The Dynamic Consultation

Pragmatics & Beyond New Series

Volume 128

The Dynamic Consultation:
A discourse analytical study of doctor–patient communication
by Marisa Cordella

The Dynamic Consultation

A discourse analytical study of doctor–patient communication

Marisa Cordella

Monash University, Australia

John Benjamins Publishing Company

Amsterdam / Philadelphia

∞™ The paper used in this publication meets the minimum requirements of American National Standard for Information Sciences – Permanence of Paper for Printed Library Materials, ANSI z39.48-1984.

Library of Congress Cataloging-in-Publication Data

Cordella, Marisa

The dynamic consultation : a discourse analytical study of doctor–patient communication / Marisa Cordella.

p. cm. (Pragmatics & Beyond, New Series, ISSN 0922-842X ; v. 128)

1. Discourse analysis. 2. Physician and patient. I. Title. II. Pragmatics & beyond ; new ser. 128.

P302.C65 2004

401'.41-dc22 2004055095

ISBN 90 272 5371 4 (Eur.) / 1 58811 558 5 (US) (Hb; alk. paper)

John Benjamins Publishing Co. · P.O. Box 36224 · 1020 ME Amsterdam · The Netherlands

John Benjamins North America · P.O. Box 27519 · Philadelphia PA 19118-0519 · USA

To Aldo

Table of contents

Preface

Communication in organizations is a major area of investigation in sociolinguistics. In the sense of "critical linguistics"[1] the structures of interaction in relevant social domains need to be made transparent. Institutions incorporate such areas and manifest power-allocations, hierarchies, systematic access to or exclusion from important positions and information, and define such fields in their subdivisions of work. Organizations have their own value-systems and narratives, which crystallize *inter alia* in ideologies unique to particular domains (Mumby 1988).

At the same time there is an important applied side to organizational research that is relevant to practice: for analyses of the status quo have made it possible to develop postulates for changes in communication patterns, for example through training programmes for members of organizations or – if we consider hospitals and doctor–patient communication – in proposals for a different approach to their clients, i.e. patients (Fiehler & Sucharowski 1992). Sociolinguistic and discourse-analytic studies have therefore proved to be an essential part of the investigation of organizations, since a purely sociological analysis is often not capable of making the details of interactive dynamics and structural processes explicit, and is therefore obliged to adopt a high level of abstraction (cf., for example, Weick 1985).

Moreover, the discourse-analytical approach has made it possible to discover the differentiated impact of explicit and latent norms and rules in discourse, and to demonstrate how structures and discursive patterns are always influential and constantly reproduced, even on the micro-levels of everyday interactions.

With few exceptions, previous research on doctor–patient communication has mostly relied on two main approaches: the medical-sociological, which is oriented towards the organization, and the linguistic, which is interested in micro-structural aspects of this communication. So far there has been little success in unifying these two aspects. For example, Aaron Cicourel (1981), using a number of case histories, already proved the advantage of a conversation-analytical procedure as opposed to quantitative psychological categorizations.

He cautions repeatedly that the structural framework must be included together with the different interests of the two principal protagonists – the doctor and the patient (doctors want to reach a diagnosis as swiftly as possible, whereas patients want to tell the story of their suffering; this results in conflicts of both time and interest ["frame-conflict"] that are sometimes difficult to resolve).

Other research has focused more and more on the analysis of individual conversational sequences, such as question–answer adjacency pairs. Since these are isolated from the context of the complete discourse, they may ultimately only be interpreted to a limited extent. Elliott Mishler, however, was able to illustrate already clearly in the 1980's that this research remained in "the voice of medicine", and that scientific interpretation was therefore done from the medical perspective, while the signals from patients were usually ignored.

The centre of interest of medical Sociology was case histories and conversations during doctors' ward-visits, however, little analysis of the conversations was provided. Nowadays, attention to health care has grown; many administrators are concerned with complaints, and the efficiency of medical systems is debated throughout many countries. The role of communication is slowly becoming acknowledged, both in written as well as spoken genres. Most importantly, the training of doctors in many countries has started to include communication skills, while taking foreign languages, translators and the problems of migrants into consideration. Moreover, the focus has also turned to gender-specific communication patterns. As recent research on communicating pain has illustrated, women and men tend to express pain in significantly different modes (Baumgartinger et al. 2002; Everts et al. 1996; Holdright & Fox 1996; Menz et al. 2002). This has had serious consequences, such as differing treatment and diagnosis.

Can a face-to-face conversation with a doctor be replaced, perhaps with new media? Could this help overcome staff shortages? On the basis of research on internet communication and on the websites of individual doctors and group practices, this kind of claim must be seen as unrealistic. The internet can only be sensibly used by those who know precisely what they are looking for. And so there are initial barriers that affect both expert knowledge and language. Medical experience is also essential, because one has to be able to distinguish between commonplace advice and detailed suggestions. If one is really looking for precise help, one inevitably comes up against specialized knowledge, scientific articles, mostly in English, on individual medical problems. How can a lay person deal with this? And how can one assess whether particular diagnoses and therapies are applicable to one? A real interaction and conversation with a doctor therefore remain indispensable. The internet or some other advisor may sometimes be helpful in finding important starting points, or in giving the feeling that others have similar problems, and thereby reducing fear and shame. Alternatively, after a proved diagnosis, it enables chat room conversations with other "fellow-sufferers", and this helps to reduce loneliness and fear. A precondition, however, must still be a conversation, not "virtual" but face-to-face. In our fast-living times, conversation and real interaction have an important value. They are increasingly relevant since they help to establish trust and to reduce a whole range of different anxieties. These two functions will become ever more important in an age of increasing uncertainty.

This is why both theoretical and empirical studies on doctor–patient communication are urgently needed. The innovative study by Marisa Cordella has succeeded in providing a very relevant and challenging interdisciplinary approach as well as a detailed empirical investigation. She has elaborated previous research in the field of (intercultural) doctor–patient communication and integrated sociological, psychological and linguistic concepts, insights and methodologies, which allow for new results. Most importantly, Cordella has made the "voices" of the patients visible while viewing the medical process as dynamic and influenced by multiple factors. Let us hope that this book reaches many readers, also practitioners in the field of medicine, and helps to trigger fruitful debates and innovative proposals for new ways of communicating with each other, in many areas of everyday life.

Ruth Wodak
June 2004

Note

1. See Lalouschek, Menz and Wodak (1990); Menz (1991); Wodak and Meyer (2001); Wodak (1996, 2004); Iedema (2003); Muntigl et al. (2000).

References

Baumgartinger, Barbara, Sator, Marlene, Binder, Ernst C., & Pobaschnig, G. (2002). Metapherngebrauch bei der Beschreibung von Brustschmerzen. *Wiener Linguistische Gazette, 70*, 45–69.

Cicourel, A. V. (1981). Language and Medicine. In Ferguson & Heath (Eds.), 403–430.

Everts, B., Karlson, B. W., Währborg, P., Hedner, T., & Herlitz, J. (1996). Localization of pain in suspected acute myocardial infarction in relation to final diagnosis, age and site and type of infarction. *Heart and Lung, 25*, 430–437.

Ferguson, Ch. & Heath, Sh. B. (Eds.). (1981). *Language in the USA*. Cambridge: Cambridge Univ. Press.

Fiehler, R. & Sucharowski, W. (Eds.). (1992). *Kommunikationsberatung und Kommunikationstraining*. Opalden: WDV.

Holdright, D. R. & Fox, K. M. (1996). Characterization and identification of women with angina pectoris. *Eur Heart J 1996, 17*, 510–517.

Iedema, R. (2003). *Post Bureaucratic Organization*. Amsterdam: Benjamins.

Lalouschek, J., Menz, F., & Wodak, R. (1990). *Alltag in der Ambulanz*. Tübingen: Narr.

Menz, F. (1991). *Der geheime Dialog*. Bern: P. Lang.

Menz, F., Lalouschek, J., Stöllberger, C., & Vodopiutz, J. (2002). Geschlechtsspezifische Unterschiede bei der Beschreibung von akutem Brustschmerz: Ergebnisse einer medizinisch-linguistischen transdisziplinären Studie. *Linguistische Berichte, 191*, 343–366.

Mishler, E. G. (1984). *The discourse of medecine*. Norwood, NJ: Ablex.

Mumby, D. K. (1988). *Communication and Power in organizations: discourse, ideology and domination*. Norwood, NJ: Ablex.

Muntigl, P., Weiss, G., & Wodak, R. (2000). *EU Discourses on Un/Employment*. Amsterdam: Benjamins.

Weick, K. (1985). *Der Prozeß des Organisierens*. Frankfurt/Main: Suhrkamp.

Wodak, R. (1996). *Disorders in Discourse*. London: Longmans.

Wodak, R. (2004). Critical Discourse Analysis. In J. Seale et al. (Eds.), *Qualitative Research Practice*. London: Sage (in press).

Wodak, R. & Meyer, M. (Eds.). (2001). *Methods of CDA*. London: Sage.

Acknowledgments

The completion of a piece of research like this requires many hours devoted entirely to the project. This devotion implies time constraints imposed upon those who are close to us, in my case my immediate family. I am grateful for the support, encouragement and constant feedback that Aldo, my friend and husband, gave me during the writing of this book. I am thankful to my daughter, Catiray, bunch of flowers, who kept me away from the computer screen or the pages of a book or article when she wanted my attention to show me her latest dance, to play her new cello piece or when she simply wanted to share with me her adolescent views of the world. This helped to keep me in touch with other realities and interests.

I wish to thank Dr. Joanne Winter for her insightful queries throughout this research, and for her comments and feedback. I am thankful to Prof. Ruth Wodak, Dr. Janet Holmes, Dr. Keith Allan and Dr. Aldo Poiani for their shrewd and useful opinions on an earlier version of this book, which have clearly enriched and improved the text presented here. My thanks are extended as well to Mr. Alun Kenwood, who read the entire first draft, for his helpful and constructive suggestions, and to Meredith Sherlock, who meticulously revised the whole text for publication.

I am grateful to Ms. Wilma Masini, who was pivotal in establishing the initial contact with the *Pontificia Universidad Católica de Chile* (PUC) in 1995–1996 and who helped to update the correct Chilean-Spanish names of the medicines mentioned in this work. I am thankful to Dr. Geoffrey Broomhall of the Monash University Clinic, who helped in revising the medical terms included in the research.

I am grateful for the *Overseas Study Program* awarded to me by the Arts Faculty of Monash University during the last semester of 2003. This grant allowed me to concentrate fully on the completion of the book.

Last but not least, I would like to give my profound thanks to Dr. Joaquín Montero, Dr. Carmen Covarrubias and Dr. Philippa Moore, who believed in this project and who allowed me to carry out the recording of doctor–patient conversations at the PUC. My sincere appreciation is extended to all the doctors and patients who cooperated in this study, as well as to the general staff of the Clinic who were always willing to lend a hand. There is no doubt that without their help this study would never have been completed.

Chapter 1

Introduction

In today's hectic world we tend to take our *good health* for granted and it is only when our body fails that health issues take centre stage, changing, sometimes dramatically, our perception of life and death.

We are all potential patients: none of us can be certain, unfortunately, that our *healthy body* will remain so indefinitely. Our visits to the doctor may be planned on a regular basis, or they can be prompted by an unexpected medical condition. Whatever the case, we are sooner or later faced with the need to communicate with a health practitioner, and the quality of this communication may be the key to assessing and managing the problem successfully.

In this book I adopt as my central tenet that good communication between doctor and patient is of vital importance for effective treatment, compliance – and (hopefully) return to health. Good communication is understood to mean both the intelligible exchange of information and the mutual recognition of the most appropriate way to participate in the exchange. In this study I describe the various discourse forms used by doctors and patients in the medical consultation as different kinds of *voices*. These *voices* are specific to the sociocultural framework of my research, but they are intended to offer a model of interaction which can be adapted and modified more widely. The model does not claim universality, but in Western societies at the end of the twentieth century, at least, tensions between the traditional disease-centred approach of bio-medical practitioners and the growing holistic expectations of their patients offer much scope for discourse analytical studies which aim to facilitate better doctor–patient communication.

My research on doctor–patient communication springs from two main interests. Firstly, studies such as this one can be used to test the hypotheses and models developed thus far, as well as to suggest new ones. In this way new approaches to the documenting, modelling and teaching of medical discourse may be developed. Secondly, I wished to identify those aspects of the talk that seemed to be particularly problematic so that special attention may be given to them when improvements in overall communication are sought. I have also been particularly concerned to analyse the participation of *both* interactants in the discourse, recognizing doctor–patient communication as a dynamic process.

The data for this study was collected in an outpatient public teaching hospital in Santiago, Chile, within the empirical framework of medical consultations of Chilean-Spanish speakers. Accordingly, the model for my research is a Chilean clinic, and medical consultations will be analysed within a specific institutional and socio-cultural paradigm. While it is not my purpose to draw on these empirical findings to establish a comparative framework, the analysis of doctor–patient communication presented here will be used to identify a set of "forms of talk" (Goffman 1981) that may occur, with linguistic, ethnic and cultural variation, elsewhere. In other words, I will argue that my findings are not unique to one socio-cultural group in one particular medical centre, but can be representative of a more general medical discourse.

In Chapter 2 I begin by exploring the existing literature from an interactional socio-linguistic perspective, incorporating both Gumperz's (1982a, 1982b, 1999) "socio-cultural background knowledge" and Goffman's (1967, 1971, 1981, 1983) "interactional framework" approaches as a way of understanding the institutional alignments and social identities that are represented in the discourse. Here both the concept of power, following Giddens's (1976, 1977, 1979, 1981, 1984, 1987) and Foucault's (1975, 1980) interpretations, and the concept of *simpatía* as a particular feature of friendly talk among Spanish speakers (following Triandis et al. 1984), are introduced. Both power and *simpatía* appear to be working together in the discourse. The chapter concludes by reviewing the medical, linguistic and sociological studies published in the area of doctor–patient communication, highlighting the major trends and findings in the field.

Chapter 3 begins with a brief review of the various approaches that have been used in the study of discourse analysis, exploring their origins and the differences between the schools of thought. The chapter then describes the research site for this project, gives a profile of the institution and the participants in the study, and documents how the data was collected. It also illustrates how doctor and patient contributions to the discourse can be deconstructed to account for their forms of talk (*voices*). The limits of the study are also discussed, in terms of the number of *voices* that are associated with each participant, and it is suggested that these could be further expanded to make finer differentiations, or reduced by using broader descriptions.

Chapters 4 to 6 then deconstruct the doctor *voices* that I have identified in the consultations: *Doctor voice* (Chapter 4), *Educator voice* (Chapter 5) and *Fellow Human voice* (Chapter 6). Chapter 7, in turn, identifies four patient *voices*:

the *voice* of *Health-related storytelling*, of *Competence*, of *Social Communicator*, and of *Initiator*. The analysis presented in these four chapters firstly observes how each *voice* can be differentiated, and discusses the discourse features commonly found in each *voice*. Chapter 8 examines the interaction of these *voices* and describes the common patterns in which they occur. I argue that switches from one *voice* to another are associated with the continual shifts of *footing* that create a dynamic relationship between doctor and patient.

Chapter 9 interprets the results of my investigation in the context of collective knowledge made available in previous studies in the field. The results are then synthesized into a *dynamic model* which takes account of the interactive processes that have been described throughout the book, and explores the performance of doctors and patients in terms of the expectations and limitations of their roles, power and knowledge. The relationships between knowledge, power and *simpatía* are discussed in light of the book's central finding that the framework of the medical consultation is one that is intrinsically asymmetrical.

Chapter 10 concludes this study by highlighting the significance of the findings and provides suggestions for future research.

CHAPTER 2

Discourse, society and doctor–patient communication

> We, however, for our part, are convinced that the chief merit of language is clearness, and we know that nothing detracts so much from this as do unfamiliar terms; accordingly we employ those terms which the bulk of people are accustomed to use . . .
>
> (Galen, *On the Natural Faculties* I.3; tr. Arthur J. Brock)

Doctor–patient communication in Western medicine has had a troubled history. Starting with Hippocrates (c. 460–380 BCE), practising physicians, who looked for natural causes of illness, were confronted with the prevalent magical thinking of their patients. This conflict between the doctor's and the patient's world views might have been at least partly resolved by better educating the patient, and yet Hippocrates' Oath reads in part:

> I will impart a knowledge of the Art to my own sons, and those of my teachers, and to disciples bound by a stipulation and oath according to the law of medicine, but to *none others.*
>
> (Hippocrates, The Oath, c. 400 BCE, tr. F. Adams, emphasis mine)

Further, Hippocrates was explicit in nominating the physician as authority figure and the consultation as an inherently unequal exchange. He stated that the onus was on the doctor to adjust his communication strategies in order to give instructions to the patient:

> . . . But whoever does not reach the capacity of the illiterate vulgar and fails to make them listen to him, misses his mark.
>
> (Hippocrates, *On Ancient Medicine*, tr. F. Adams)

The Roman doctor and writer Galen (129 – c. 210 CE), who spent several years as physician to the gladiators in Pergamum, continued the scientific tradition of Hippocrates; in the Middle Ages the tradition was kept alive by Islamic scholars such as ibn Sina, also known as Avicenna, and ibn Rushd, Averroes. The prevailing mechanistic view of medicine and medical practice took shape in the Renaissance, when modern science was born and scholars devoted to medical research framed the human body as a machine. Two influential medical works of this period have the suggestive titles *De Humani Corporis Fabrica* (Andreas Vesalius 1543) and *De Motu Cordis* (William Harvey 1628). Although this bio-medical approach did indeed spark the enormous revolution in medical science that is continuing in our own time, it de-emphasized the role of communication in the work of healing.

Be that as it may, doctors and their patients find themselves engaged in a discourse in which the manner whereby the technical information is conveyed may be as important as the information itself. The aim of this study is to show, through analysis of recorded data, how doctors and patients actually communicate in the modern clinical setting and how their forms of talk may either help or hinder the patient's understanding and co-operation. An interactional socio-linguistic approach has been adopted that incorporates Gumperz's (1982a, 1982b, 1999) "socio-cultural background knowledge" and Goffman's (1967, 1971, 1981, 1983) "interactional framework". The theories of these two scholars complement each other in developing an integrated framework of language, society and culture; and in the context of the medical consultation they can help to shed light on the different alignments of doctor and patient that account for their different roles and contributions in the exchange. Because this study argues that the medical consultation is an asymmetrical event, the concept of *power* will be discussed as it has been developed in the areas of social theory and critical discourse analysis. Because the research for this study was undertaken in a Chilean clinic, the concept of *simpatía* in discourse is also introduced appropriately here.

In order to set the medical discourse presented here in its socio-cultural context, the linguistic features found in everyday and institutional conversations are described, followed by a brief discussion of micro and macro realities; I suggest that the performance realized in a micro setting (i.e. the consultation) is unlikely to be independent of socio-cultural relationships at the macro level. For example, the exercise of power is not necessarily peculiar to the medical consultation, but may be representative of an asymmetrical interaction in discourses of other social contexts as well.

In this chapter I also offer an introduction to the two most prevalent medical approaches (namely, bio-medical and socio-relational), identifying the linguistic studies that have contributed to the understanding of doctor–patient communication as reflecting either an emphasis on the body part to be fixed or on the patient to be treated. The asymmetrical qualities of the consultation may be considered in light of the particular model or approach adopted in the interaction. Finally, the literature on doctor–patient communication is surveyed, looking at both the medical and linguistic approaches to the subject and arguing for a synthesis of both. The importance of sociological variables in medical discourse, such as age, class and gender, is also discussed.

2.1 A multi-disciplinary approach: Interactional socio-linguistics

Interactional socio-linguistics is a multi-disciplinary field of research that combines anthropological, sociological and linguistic studies with the aim of understanding and interpreting the relationships between culture, society and language. Gumperz, as a linguist–anthropologist, and Goffman, as a sociologist, have been pivotal in this field in giving shape to a comprehensive conception of language and society. Gumperz's interest focuses on the concept of language as a means of social interaction. When people come together in a conversation they not only exchange words, but also, in the course of talking, recreate socio-cultural knowledge; in this process they reproduce a network of relationships that is identified either implicitly or explicitly in their verbal behaviour.

During the verbal exchange, both inferences and contextual cues play a fundamental role in the speakers' interpretative schema and therefore in the comprehension of the speech (Gumperz 1971, 1982a, 1999). The hearer interprets what the speaker *means to say* by drawing inferences from what is *actually said*. The speaker's analogous interpretation of the same act reflects the participants' shared social background knowledge necessary for a correct reading of the contextual cues. Thus, what is said and how it is said do not occur in a vacuum, but are the result of each speaker's intention to convey particular information that expresses both communicative competence in the language as well as the socio-cultural background (speaker's speech community) of that information. Various discourse strategies are used to achieve this (Gumperz & Hymes 1972). In order to make this point clearer, I have selected one of the examples offered by Gumperz, based on his socio-linguistic studies carried out in North America.[1] Following a graduate seminar, an African-American student approaches his white instructor and asks for an appointment.

a. Could I talk to you for a minute? I'm gonna apply for a fellowship and I was wondering if I could get a recommendation?

The instructor replied:

b. O.K. Come along to the office and tell me what you want to do.

As the instructor and the rest of the group left the room, the black student said, turning his head ever so slightly to the other students:

c. Ahma git me a gig! (Rough gloss: "I'm going to get myself some support.") (Gumperz 1982a: 30)

Gumperz presents this example to show how individuals make inferences about someone else's speech. He asked a group of students what they understood about this exchange. The interpretation varied depending on the individual's socio-cultural knowledge and contact with the African-American community. For example, the last utterance "Ahma git me a gig!" was interpreted as a shift from the standard English usage of (a) to the African-American English of (c) by those whose knowledge of African-American speech was minimal. The interpretation given by African-Americans and white individuals who had greater exposure to African-American speakers was that the utterance was an African-American speaker's identity marker. When the African-American speaker asked for a recommendation letter from a white American instructor he used a form of talk that conformed to the one predominantly in use in white society. The identity marker was used in communication with his peers.

This passage exemplifies Gumperz's theory of language in interaction, and serves to illustrate the framework for this present research. Firstly, a theory of interaction is based on the shared knowledge of speaker and hearer of both the language and the social rules. This shared knowledge has to be such as to at least permit common understanding, and must take into account the underlying expectations of each participant; that is, the interpretative frame or schema of the situation. As Tannen (1993: 14–15) has observed:

> The only way we can make sense of the world is to see the connections between things, and between present things we have experienced before or heard about. These vital connections are learned as we grow up and live in a given culture.

There is therefore a culturally determined propensity to perceive and assimilate what makes sense and is recognizable to our mind (Gumperz 1982a: 13). Following van Dijk, the notion of schema needs to be understood at the level of social cognition, thus:

a. Structures and strategies of social information in memory, for instance, about groups, functionally reflect the role of this information in communication and interaction, and

b. These processes of communication and interaction are structurally embedded in social micro and macro contexts. These two dimensions assign

> both a functional and a contextual dimension to the nature of social cognition. (van Dijk 1987:251–252)

This implies, according to van Dijk, that people process social information as members of a social group rather than as separate, unconnected individuals.

Secondly, Gumperz's example above highlights the concept of inference and the importance of socio-cultural background knowledge for an understanding of contextual cues. Thirdly, it highlights the individual's ability to acquire a repertoire of varieties of the language, as well as the social skills for knowing when it is appropriate (or effective) to use one form or another. According to Gumperz (1982a:34):

> The use of one variety where another is expected is not simply an instance of inappropriate usage, but can have communicative significance.

Whereas for Gumperz socio-cultural background knowledge has an effect on the understanding and production of an utterance, for Goffman (1971, 1981) language reflects the social roles and relationships that people negotiate throughout an encounter. In this next section I summarize Goffman's contribution to interactional socio-linguistics.

Initially Goffman's idea was to create a field of research separate from sociology, claiming that the study of interaction, what he called "interaction order", was a field of research in its own right (Goffman 1981). His work at first appeared to be carried out unconventionally; according to Drew and Wotton (1988:2), "no clear hypotheses, no standard research designs, nor even a theory that could be tested or used to make sense of a variety of research findings" were presented. One of the biggest complaints about Goffman's work has been that his research is not empirical (Levinson 1988: 162) and it is difficult to see how it could be so. In other words, in contrast with Gumperz, Goffman's models are not based on ethnographic research but on the social framework of any conversation; indeed, Randall (1988: 52), speaks of Goffman's "ecological" perspective, since his stance is one of observing what people do and say when they are in the presence of others. It has also been said that his research has methodological flaws. Drew and Wotton, for example, mention vagueness in the use of concepts, lack of care in managing the data, and subjective data selection.

All of these observations may have diminished the initial impact of Goffman's ideas and views of a participation framework of interaction. However, his contribution to the field of interactional socio-linguistics was profoundly increased in his later years when he became associated with the University of Pennsylvania, and when his research began to be influenced by colleagues in the fields of anthropology and sociology making an impact in linguistics. Goffman realized the importance of studying face-to-face interactions and of carrying out micro-analysis to better understand the "traffic of rules" that makes the interactions possible in the first place. In his own words:

> My concern over the years has been to promote acceptance of this face-to-face domain as an analytically viable one – a domain which might be titled, for want of any happy name, the *interaction order* – a domain whose preferred method of study is microanalysis. (Goffman 1983: 2)

The interaction order has been defined by Goffman as the "syntactical relationships" (1967: 2) that exist among individuals acting in the presence of others. For him, participants exert mutual influence over each other when they are in near proximity to each other:

> An interaction may be defined as all the interaction which occurs throughout any one occasion when a given set of individuals are in one another's continuous presence. (Goffman 1959: 26)

This implies that the concept of interaction for Goffman includes not only the production of language but every other action carried out by participants as well. He defines the "interdependency of action" (1963: 22) that enables the interaction to occur. In the presence of others, the individual performs a role associated with a given situation, and this always affects the performance of other participants in the encounter.

When an individual (e.g. a doctor) performs a role to the same audience (e.g. a patient) on different occasions (e.g. different consultation times) a social relationship is likely to result. A social role is defined by Goffman as:

> The enactment of rights and duties attached to a given status ... we can say that a social role will involve one or more parts and that each of these different parts may be presented by the performer on a series of occasions to the same kinds of audience or to an audience of the same persons. (1959: 27)

During the consultation, doctors play the social role of care providers whose duties and obligations are attached to their medical profession and enacted during their interaction with the patient.

In any given encounter, individuals gather information from each other in two different ways:

a. Participants *give* content information. The individual who provides the information supplies the content of the delivered message through the use of symbolic actions (including language) that are reciprocally recognized as being external to the speaker him/herself.

b. Individuals also *give off* additional information. This relates to the complementary information that the recipient obtains from the speaker's choice of words, linguistic features (intonation, speed of delivery, etc.), body language and so on – idioms that are inseparable from the speaker. This additional information can have an effect on the meaning attached to the transmitted message.

Thus, both the information delivered and the form of the message may have an impact on the interaction order. This in turn may alter the syntactical relationship of the speakers and cause a shift in the participation structure. This shift is referred to as *footing* and this is now discussed below.

2.1.1 Footing

Goffman took an interest in the work of Gumperz (1971) who observed that code switching may not necessarily be associated with the shift from one language to another, but with changes in the participants' behaviour and the position they occupy in the discourse. This is what Goffman refers to as the participant's stance and alignment in the encounter (see Giddens's "dialectic of control", p. 15 below). Goffman's concept of *footing* (1981) is based on his conviction that the dyadic division of speaker/hearer is not sufficient to understand the participation framework of an interaction. He argues that speakers may use different forms of talk depending on their alignment in a given context. For example:

> ... we can momentarily affect a podium speech register, or provide a theatrical version (burlesqued, melodramatic) of an aside. All of which, of course, provides extra warrant – indeed, perhaps, the main warrant – for differentiating various participation frameworks in the first place. (1981: 154)

A theatrical performance is Goffman's most descriptive illustration of the different social masks that we as individuals wear in everyday encounters. Any shift from one form of talk to another constitutes an example of footing and it is precisely at this point, as Goffman emphasizes, that footing is shown to be "very commonly language-linked" (1981: 128). In order to identify shifts in the participation structure of individuals, Goffman centres his attention on footing and underlines the main characteristics of this term:

a. "Participant's alignment, or set, or stance, or posture, or projected self is somehow at issue".

b. The participant's performance cannot be entirely traced back to grammatical sentences; however "it seems clear that a cognitive unit of some kind is involved, minimally, perhaps a 'phonemic clause'. Prosodic, not syntactic, segments are implied".

c. A continuum of stances needs to be observed: these can range from extremely subtle to clearly perceivable shifts of footing.

d. Footing generally involves participants' code switching and/or slight changes in tone of voice, volume, rhythm and pitch, among other sound markers.

e. "The bracketing of a 'higher level' phase or episode of interaction is commonly involved, the new footing having a liminal role, serving as a buffer between two more substantially sustained episodes". (1981: 128)

Even the slightest change in one participant's language and behaviour can alter the stance of the other(s) and create a new alignment in the exchange. This shift from one footing to another can then determine the participation structure of the interaction that follows.

Participants in a verbal exchange often perform a number of roles, which Goffman differentiates as *animator*, *author* and *principal* (1981: 167; see also Bakhtin's description of dialogic voices in Holquist 1981; Morris 1994). The *animator* has the role of emitting the right sounds to produce a recognizable utterance. This is not a social but a functional role, one which we might term the "machine of communication-production". The *author* is defined as the individual who authors a text that is scripted and formulated. *Principals* establish a position by conveying personal beliefs and commitments in their own words. The principal represents an active individual "in some particular social identity or role, some special capacity as a member of a group, office, category, relationship, association, or whatever, some socially based source of self-identification" (Goffman 1981: 144–145). Following Goffman, one person can perform all three roles simultaneously or in any combination of one or more roles during the interaction.

In a hospital consultation both the doctor and the patient will be animating their own words through talk and in this process will be scripting (authoring) a text. In addition they will convey an individual social identity through their projection of beliefs and commitments (as principals) in the course of the exchange. Any shift from one form of talk to another can be interpreted as a change in the stance and alignment of participants that will affect the further contributions that each makes to the discourse. This leads us then to a consideration of *power*, both as it operates in conversations between individuals and as a reflection of the hierarchical system of the social group.

2.2 Power, society and discourse

Much of the research undertaken in critical discourse analysis has been centred on the exercise of power and on the different participation of individuals in a context in which power imbalance comes into play (Ainsworth-Vaughn 1994, 1998; Borges 1986; Fairclough 1985, 1989, 1992; Fisher 1991; Fisher & Todd 1983, 1986a; Holmes et al. 1999; Tannen 1987; Todd & Fisher 1993; van Dijk 1995a, 1995b, 1996, 1997b; Wodak 1989, 1996, 1999b; Wodak & Matouschek 1993). Following Tannen (1987:5), power can be interpreted as an activity that separates those *knowledgeable* from those *not knowledgeable* within the social system. Those who know the system are doing

> Business as-usual on their home turf, while their clients pass through the system, often confused and always ignorant of the intricacies of the system.

This asymmetry emerges as the central issue when trying to comprehend the exercise of power in the exchange. Investigators have placed particular emphasis on the institutional and societal context of an asymmetrical interaction; and the dialectic between the exercise of power and the discourse constraints that differentiate participants of unequal power has been the concern of critical discourse analysts whose interest in "uncovering injustice, inequality, talking sides with powerless and suppressed" (Wodak 1989:xiv) has been the core motivation of their studies.

My intention in documenting dominant behaviour in doctor–patient relationships is not to focus on only those instances of injustice and/or inequalities that may occur, but rather to understand the expression of power as one form of talk that interacts with other forms of talk in medical discourse. Following Davis (1988:86):

> Although power cannot be eliminated from a study of interaction, this does not mean that it is sufficient for explaining how social interaction is produced.

Accordingly, I expect to find different expressions of power interacting in doctor–patient communication. I have confined the discussion of power in this study to those theoretical features that can contribute to our understanding of an institutional interaction such as the medical one; however, I hope to be able to offer some insights into the broader inter-relationship of power and society, and the connection between power and discourse. The conceptual ideas of Foucault (1975, 1980) and Giddens (1976, 1977, 1979, 1981, 1984, 1987) are taken into account in my analysis, and their ideas will be expanded on with contributions developed in critical discourse analysis.

Foucault does not describe power as a colossal force that oppresses a particular group of individuals, a social body that dictates the "universality of will" (1980:55). On the contrary, power is perceived as not being in anyone's hands.

> Power must [be] analysed as something that circulates, or rather as something which only functions in the form of a chain. It is never localised here or there, never in anybody's hands, never appropriated as a commodity or piece of wealth. (1980:98)

In Foucault's view, power must be seen as a fluid activity that is exerted or suffered by individuals in a dynamic way.

> Power is employed and exercised through a net-like organization. And not only do individuals circulate between its threads; they are always in the position of simultaneously undergoing and exercising this power. They are not only its inert or consenting target; they are always also the elements of its circulation. In other words, individuals are the vehicles of power, not its points of application. (1980:98)

He does not perceive power as a crushing force that operates at a supra-individual level, but rather as a force that can be generated from *within* the individual. This implies that power is exercised through the individual's actions (1980:89). Further, Foucault offers an alternative way of interpreting power as a positive energy. He writes:

> What makes power hold good, what makes it accepted, is simply the fact that it doesn't only weigh on us as a force that says no, but that it traverses and produces things, it induces pleasure, forms knowledge, produces discourse. It needs to be considered as a productive network which runs through the whole social body, much more than as a negative instance whose function is repression. (1980:119)

That is, power need not be a destructive and stifling energy but can produce a creative network of relationships that engage individuals within a social group.

One of Foucault's limitations, according to Wodak (1996), has been that *agency* is not included in Foucault's thinking about power, unlike Giddens, who sees "an intrinsic relation between agency and power" (1979:6). Giddens's theory of the exercise of power develops around "the capability of the actor to intervene in a series of events so as to alter their course" (Giddens 1976:11).

His work, mainly his structuration theory, stems from considerations of how power operates at the level of social practice, recognizing that the dynamic organization of society has its roots in the inter-relationship of time and space (Giddens 1976, 1979). For Giddens, time is an essential part of social action. The concept of time in relation to the production of a discourse is also considered a fundamental component by Wodak (1995, 1996, 1999a) and Fairclough and Wodak (1997). They refer to this as "intertextuality", positing that the discourse exists always in relation to another discourse occurring at a particular point in time (either synchronically or diachronically). In other words, while each medical consultation is unique, it will also share some similarities with those in the past and/or the future and with current discourses of the societal group as a reflection of existing or emergent social practices.

According to Tannen, the dynamism of discourse is also influenced by changes in the interaction itself. She suggests that "power may be there in different forms and in different ways – all constantly changing in dynamic response to the behaviour of others" (1987: 5). The dynamic composition of power relates to Giddens's theory of structuration that centres on the *action* that is accomplished in an exchange. In his view, society works as follows:

> A. One: *Sociology is not concerned with a "pre-given" universe of objects, but with one which is constituted or produced by the active doings of subjects.*
> A. Two: *The production and reproduction of society thus has to be treated as a skilled performance on the part of its members.*
> (Giddens's emphasis, 1976: 160)

Following Giddens, individuals are perceived as adept and knowledgeable agents who are able "to monitor their activities at various concurrent flows" (1976: 83) because, as social actors, they are *aware* of the demands of any given situation. This view relates to the active role that the individual may play in social practice by bringing changes to the course of the event, even in the most adverse circumstances, through a "dialectic of control" (Giddens 1981, 1987). This dynamic idea of interaction is referred to as "duality of structure"; that is, structures are both created and recreated through individuals' actions.

> Language exists as a "structure", syntactical and semantic, only in so far as there are some kind of traceable consistencies in what people say, in the speech acts which they perform. From this aspect, to refer to rules of syntax, for example, is to refer to the reproduction of "like elements"; on the other hand, such rules also *generate* the totality of speech-acts which is the spoken language. It is this dual structure, as both inferred from observations of human doings, and yet as also operating as a medium whereby those doings are made

> possible, that has to be grasped through the notions of structuration and reproduction. (Giddens's emphasis, 1976: 121–122)

Hence, the reproduction of a structure is both the means of social practice and the medium through which social practices are preserved in time. Nonetheless, the exercise of *dialectic of control* has the potential to make alterations to those structures, much in the same way as, in the process of reproduction – following a biological analogy –, changes such as mutations may occur. In terms of social theory, actors/agents are capable of changing structures in the process of reproducing them. While rules exist, they are in a state of constant transformation.

The perception of power as a transformative and non-static activity is further explored by Wodak (1989, 1996, 1999a) in her work in critical discourse analysis. She believes there is a need to understand both where (institutional setting) and how (participants' interaction) power is produced in order to find alternatives to deal with it or to resist it. "'*Diagnosis' first, interpretation and 'therapy' to follow!*" (Wodak's emphasis, 1989: xiv). This suggests that once there is an understanding of how power is exercised in a particular context, there is a chance of bringing changes into social practice.

Communication in institutions appears to be a fertile ground for the reproduction of power because participants of different status come face-to-face in a system where resources are not equally distributed (Fairclough 1989, 1992; Giddens 1976, 1987; van Dijk 1995a, 1995b, 1997b). Giddens's early work (1977) describes the concept of power in relation to the resources available to individuals and to the rules that structure, give shape and organize social practice. Rules, their dynamic nature notwithstanding, are followed by individuals as a collective norm and are therefore sanctioned by society (Giddens 1979). They thus present as a double-sided and paradoxical phenomenon: they both enable and constrain the exercise of power. As such, they relate "to the constitution of meaning, and that [relates] to sanctions involved in social conduct" (1979: 82, borrowing from Foucault).

Social sanctions vary in severity and can range from the most violent response to the absence of any talk (Giddens 1984: 178). According to Giddens, social interaction is more than a set of rules that must be followed in a given context, since the outcome of an interaction is affected by the resources available to individuals. The distribution of resources separates people from one another when the "resources are asymmetrically distributed ... [and] members are seldom really peers in the interaction game" (Davis 1988: 87). Nevertheless, this does not mean that an asymmetrical interaction necessarily leaves one of the participants without the opportunity of exercising some power over the other. In Giddens's view any agent can transform the course of an event. Davis (1988: 88) highlights the connection between power and agency:

> By linking power to agency, it becomes essential to uncover the subtle mix of what actors do (and refrain from doing), what they achieve (and fail to achieve) and what they might have done (but didn't).

Giddens's notion of power has not passed uncriticized by linguists working within his model of social theory. According to Davis, the theory describes only generalized features of power, leaving unattended a clear definition of actors/agents as well as a definition that could account for the use of rules and resources. Davis also argues that Giddens does not identify the contextual phenomena that organize power in social practice. She writes:

> Power relations are always and everywhere contextual. They are embedded in *specific* contexts, involving *specific* actors or groups of actors drawing upon *specific* rules and resources which are organized in *specifically* structured ways. Power, along with structures of domination, is implicated in concrete situated social practices. (Davis's emphasis, 1988: 99)

The specificity of the context and the involvement of actors/agents have been widely recognized as vital components of discourse and power (Davis 1988; Holmes et al. 1999; Todd & Fisher 1993; Wodak 1996, 1999b). Although Giddens's abstract framework presents some obstacles to his theory, his work has been widely used by social analysts to interpret the inter-relationship of power, agency and society (see Craib 1992 for criticism and commentaries).

An alternative view of the notion of power is presented by van Dijk, whose interpretation is rooted in the power/control that elitist groups (such as politicians and journalists) exercise over less powerful groups (such as ordinary citizens). He notes that "one group has power over another group if it has some form of control over the other group" (1997b: 17). Similarly, "power is not simply imposed, but often shared and distributed over several powerful groups" (1997b: 23). Control over a group of people can be manifested by making them act, or restraining them from acting, in accordance with what is desired by the control group. The ways in which people are made to do what the powerful group wants vary in terms of both the force of repression and the discourse strategies used to achieve desired ends. Van Dijk notes that although coercive power (e.g. military force) can be imposed to make a group adopt a certain behaviour, most of the time the power exercised over a societal group is mental (cognitive). Thus cognition appears to be one of the three key elements in van Dijk's notion of power/control, the other two being discourse and action. He states:

> Mind control and the actions that derive from it may be based on even more subtle and indirect forms of text and talk. Instead of letting others know what we want through commands, requests, suggestions or advice, we may shape their minds in such a way that they will act as we want out of their own free will. (1997b: 19)

This mental manipulation stays unrecognized by the individual who becomes the target of it. Van Dijk refers to this as "hegemonic power" because it makes people behave "as if it were natural, normal, or simply a consensus. No commands, requests or even suggestions are necessary" (1997b: 19). Hence, hegemonic power shapes people's minds in order to make them do what the dominant group wishes. This control is achieved through discourse, albeit "subtle and indirect", which, when unchallenged, produces a cognitive appreciation of an event, over time, by targeted individuals. Thus for van Dijk (1997b: 24):

> Social power of groups is not monolithic, permanent or without contradictions. It is daily being exercised and enacted by group members, also through text and talk. Such individual enactment allows for variation, dissent and even change, which also partly explains historical changes of power.

By focusing in this section on definitions of power as it is produced and reproduced through discourse within the social group, we can now summarize the main features relating to the concept of power that will recur throughout this study:

1. Discourse reproduces power, and power is maintained through discourse.
2. Power is contextualized both in time and place.
3. Power is not a faceless energy but operates through an individual's actions.
4. Power is exercised in a dynamic way by actors/agents who can alter the course of an event.
5. Power is both enabling and constraining.

2.2.1 Discourse, power and *simpatía*

If in the medical consultation we encounter different forms of talk, we may wish to ask whether all forms of talk are associated with the exercise of power or whether there are some that allow an alternative interpretation.

Previous studies have identified that the *blunt* form of power is not always present in medical discourse. For example, Davis notes in her study that "control was not accomplished in a straightforward fashion ... but rather in a paradoxically friendly and even intimate fashion" (1988: 283). Fisher and Todd (1986) recorded a similar pattern of behaviour when male doctors were talking to their female patients in relation to methods of contraception. But this interpretation still has power at its core. In other words, the above studies found that power is always present in the interaction and only the way it is exercised varies from an authoritarian and coercive form to a more subtle, gentle and presumably palatable mode.

An alternative view to the central role of power can be found in Erzinger (1989, 1991), who focused on the misunderstandings that arose between Spanish speakers and non-Spanish speakers interacting with doctors whose level of Spanish varied from near-native to poor. She found that problems of communication arose mainly because of a mismatch of communication styles resulting from cultural differences. Erzinger explored the concept of *simpatía*, as studied by Triandis et al. in social psychology, who define it as follows:

> [*Simpatía*] has no equivalent in English but refers to a permanent personal quality where an individual is perceived as likeable, attractive, fun to be with, and easygoing ... behaves with dignity and respect towards others, and seems to strive for harmony in interpersonal relations. This latter characteristic implies a general avoidance of interpersonal conflict and a tendency for positive behaviors to be emphasised in positive situations and negative behaviors to be deemphasised in negative situations. (1984: 1363)

Erzinger notes that *simpatía* is a cultural quality that can only be defined through illustration, but it is manifested through conversational style as well as supportive gestures that are used to favour a co-operative interaction in which both participants can understand each other. Although there were instances in Erzinger's study where conflict did emerge, there were also occasions in which tensions between doctor and patient were demonstrably avoided through the use of *simpatía*. The avoidance of unpleasantness (criticizing, fighting, insulting) in asymmetrical exchanges has also been documented in a study carried out in Santiago de Chile by Katie Forbes and the author (Forbes & Cordella 1999). Importantly, it has also been observed that playful argumentative style can be interpreted in Chilean-Spanish as a way of showing camaraderie and friendship in the interaction (Cordella & Forbes 1998).

Cordella (1999) performed a preliminary study to evaluate the presence of *simpatía* in the medical discourse of Chilean-Spanish speakers and found examples of discourse strategies employed by the doctor that were designed to make the conversation friendlier, such as an *in crescendo* informal greeting, respectful language, allowing the patient time to answer, latching (see p. 56 below), avoiding jargon, and choosing colloquialisms. Is *simpatía* simply a *nice* way to exercise persuasive power, or is it something else? This issue will be addressed in the current study.

Before starting to analyse the forms of talk that doctors and patients employ when they interact and identifying the discourse functions associated with these forms, I make a distinction between discourse used in an institutional (medical) setting and discourse used in everyday talk.

2.3 Everyday and institutional talk

People typically engage in a number of conversations during the day. The type of conversation (between friends, co-workers, parents and children, doctors and patients), the medium or channel of communication (telephone, internet, face-to-face) and the nature of the exchange (a greeting, lecture, instruction, medical visit) all determine how the speech is modulated. As well as providing the *content* (what is said or done) of the conversation, speakers portray both the *social relation* they bring to the discourse and the *subject position* they occupy in the speech (Fairclough 1989:46). In short, communication is conditioned by a number of variables that stipulate certain social expectations as to how the discourse should be performed.

For example, let us follow the "discourse track" of an ordinary person during a typical day. Our imaginary individual has an afternoon appointment with a specialist doctor. In the morning she has stopped at a petrol station and exchanged some words with the cashier. She has then gone to work and spoken briefly with colleagues. Later in the day this person has chaired an executive meeting where important issues have been discussed, and in the afternoon she has undergone a number of medical tests and has developed a conversation with several specialists to determine a diagnosis. In each of these communicative events the content of the talk will be different and the individual will most probably have presented a different social relation and subject position on each occasion. Her speech will have taken on differential discourse indicators and modulations appropriate to each event.

According to Goffman (1981), *everyday talk* consists of a conversation that does not seek an elevated role or require any special competency in order to be carried out successfully. Indeed, even the simplest gesture may suffice to accomplish an everyday performance. A similar view is taken by Prieto-Castillo (1999), who emphasizes that the knowledge required to engage in everyday talk does not need to be a specialized one. In "ordinary conversation" (Fisher & Todd 1986) there is no need to show a theoretical appreciation of a current affair or a state of being, for example. Nonetheless, Prieto-Castillo claims that everyday talk does require the speaker to respond promptly to the demands placed upon the speech (1999:38), which include knowledgeable use of the turn-taking system (Sacks et al. 1974) and communication strategies bound to the socio-cultural group. For Prieto-Castillo, the realization of everyday talk achieves both a functional goal, like asking someone to do something, and the interpersonal satisfaction that arises from conversation for its own sake: *para gozar con el acto mismo de la comunicación* (1999:41) ("to enjoy the act of communication itself"). Further, everyday talk is a versatile form of language that allows the pleasurable indulgence of "playing with words" in order to show friendship and warmth towards others. Fairclough (1992) uses the term "conversationalism" to refer to friendly talk (the use of feedback that conveys attentiveness and expressions of empathy). Conversationalism may have been present in our imaginary medical consultation above.

Fisher and Todd observe that, when a discourse is studied as a social activity, there are considerable similarities in the performance of the speakers. They identify everyday talk as having discourse patterns that are recurrent in conversations:

> There is an expectation of balanced participation which is, in most cases, realized. Speakers take turns and change topics in orderly fashion. They ask and answer questions, exchange greetings, and interrupt each other in equal measure. (1986:ix)

In *institutional conversations*, by contrast, the basis is laid for other kinds of discourse patterns that bespeak an unequal exchange. Here the "balanced participation" of everyday talk is replaced by an interaction that is inherently asymmetrical. On the one hand, there are the insiders (those with knowledge of the system) and, on the other, the outsiders (those with little or no knowledge of the system). As Fisher and Todd (1986:ix) observe:

> This asymmetry is highlighted in institutional contexts. The structure of the institution is organized so as to lend those in power the authority to pursue defined goals. This authority is reflected in the forms and functions (structure and content) of educational, legal and medical discourse.

The medical institution has been described as acting as a *gate-keeper* in this regard (Erickson & Shultz 1982; Royster 1990) and Parsons (1951) has suggested that doctor–patient interactions are *essentially* asymmetrical. Doctors who are familiar with the hospital or clinic and its procedures are able to make decisions regarding their patient's health, whereas patients enter the consultation as outsiders and are sometimes unaware of the medical procedures that will be involved in their treatment. This difference marks the first asymmetry of the medical relationship and it is present even before the interaction takes place. Further, the roles (social relations) of doctor and patient are clearly prescribed – to the doctor's advantage: the doctor has been trained for his/her specialist position while patients seldom present with any expertise in their role as "patient". Wodak (1996:2) observes that *disorders in discourse* and other communication problems may occur for these very reasons:

> From gaps between distinct and insufficiently coincident cognitive worlds: the gulfs that separate insiders from outsiders, members of institutions from clients of those institutions, and elites from normal citizens uninitiated in the arcana of bureaucratic language and life.

According to Maynard, medical discourse presents features of asymmetry which are "not so in any unadulterated, comprehensive, or totalistic fashion, but in particular and specifiable ways" (1991:485). If this asymmetry is challenged, the result is the so-called *frame conflict*, in which

> Worlds of knowledge and interests collide with one another, and those who possess linguistic as well as institutional power invariably prevail.
> (Wodak 1996:2)

The socio-cultural realities expressed in the micro situation of the medical consultation reproduce an *organized* institutional interaction within the individual discourse. Conversely, the macro societal levels of the socio-cultural groups are projected and consolidated through the specific discourse of the institution. The differential alignment of doctor and patient in the medical consultation requires each participant to *rehearse* their social roles, and this in turn tends to reinforce, maintain and perpetuate their subject position. This inter-relation more broadly has been a fertile field of research for sociologists and critical discourse analysts. The following section will develop this point further.

2.4 Micro and macro realities of a socio-cultural group

Sociological research (e.g. Grimshaw 1981; Molotch & Boden 1985) suggests that the production of talk is inexorably linked to context in its broadest sense:

> The organization of talk is tied to social structure generally – to the political, economic and historic forces of which talk is inevitably part.
> (Molotch & Boden 1985:273)

Following Wodak (1995:206), language and the social are "connected to each other through a dialectical relationship", which interpretation takes into account the dynamic social processes that are historically based (Wodak 1995, 1996, 1999a). Thus, the understanding of talk requires an interpretative perspective on the *social structure* that makes the talk relevant and identifiable to other speakers, including recognition of the communication constraints and obligations imposed in different socio-historical situations (Gumperz & Hymes 1972). This implies that the micro level (such as a medical consultation) needs to be understood in relation to the macro level of the socio-cultural group in which the consultation takes place. The content of the speech and the social relations and subject positions of the participants can be interpreted as a micro performance which is not unique to that particular event, but is rather representative of similar performances that, taken together, reflect the social interactions across the broader (macro) organizational sphere.

Discourse analysis and critical analysis research (Cicourel 1975, 1981, 1995; Fairclough 1985, 1989, 1992, 1995; Fisher & Groce 1985, 1990; Holmes 1990, 1997; Holmes et al. 1999; Todd & Fisher 1993; van Dijk 1987, 1996, 1997a, 1997b; Wodak 1989, 1996, 1999a, 1999b) account for the accomplishment of participants' speech by analysing discourse as an interactive phenomenon in which both *social structure* and *social interaction* are involved. Fisher and Groce describe *social structure* as the "relationship between interaction and institutional, structural and cultural forces" (1990:225). This suggests that discourse has a dynamic relationship with the macro level of operation in which socio-cultural expectations are likely to be reciprocated:

> By treating social interaction and social structure as reflexively related, features of a larger social structure ... can be found in the analysis of talk, whereas the act of talking reveals this structure and displays how talking helps to sustain it.
> (Fisher & Groce 1990:225)

Doctor and patient communication has been studied in the fields of discourse analysis and critical analysis as a discourse that reflects social, political, historical and cultural aspects. It is *social* because it occurs as a face-to-face interaction; it is *political* because it reflects the power imbalances of a hierarchical organization (Fisher & Groce 1990; Molotch & Boden 1985; Todd & Fisher 1993; Waitzkin 1983; Wodak 1996, 1999b); it is *historical* because it may show changes (e.g. institutional and interrelational) over time (Fairclough & Wodak 1997; Fisher & Todd 1986; Helman 1994; Wodak 1999a); and finally it is *cultural* because socio-cultural values and beliefs emerge in the interaction (Andary et al. 2003; Fisher 1991; Fisher & Groce 1990; Hein & Wodak

1987; Kleinman 1980; Pollard & Hyatt 1999; van Dijk 1997a, 1997b; Wodak 1996, 1999b).

The approach used in this study seeks to understand the medical exchange at two levels: the micro and the macro. The micro level accounts for the discourse sequences and the use of particular communication strategies that are accomplished through face-to-face interactions. The macro level attempts to:

a. Find explanations for the participants' forms of talk in the context of the medical institution and the social/cultural constraints operating on individuals, and
b. Understand the causal link between the interaction and "macro-institutional factors": for example, the differential understanding of health issues at the socio-cultural level; the medical practices, procedures and treatments adopted in a given institution or society.

In summary, the consultation itself is not performed in a vacuum, independent of other discourses and divorced from socio-temporal realities – including global structures and supra-systems (such as the internet) that may have an impact on communication, relationships and health care (Welch Cline 2003). Similarly, we should not overlook the impact that one particular medical approach may have when it is favoured over another in the consultation. In the next section I will review the two most widely used approaches in Western medicine, emphasizing the main characteristics that distinguish the *bio-medical* from the *socio-relational* as they affect the interaction between doctors and their patients.

2.5 Bio-medical and socio-relational approaches to doctor–patient communication

Western medicine and its associated discourse tend to operate within a *bio-medical* framework whose reductionist approach views health primarily as a biological phenomenon (Mishler 1984). As such, it tends to favour an asymmetrical relationship between doctor and patient, with the doctor mostly seeking information about the patient's complaint, giving a diagnosis and prescribing a treatment. According to Mishler, medical training has tended to stress the

> Technical–scientific skills and the diagnosis of specific diseases; rather than the patient being viewed as a person, the person is viewed as a patient. (1984:9)

This emphasis on the body part that needs to be "patched up" means that the effect of the illness on the whole life of the patient may be overlooked. Practitioners who adopt the *socio-relational* framework, on the other hand, aim to engage in the patient's "lifeworld" (Mishler 1984) by being a good listener and using the patient's own life experiences to build up the discourse. Mishler suggests that a patient-centred approach is more "humane" as it shows:

> Respect for the dignity of patients as persons and recognition of their problems within the context of their lifeworld of meaning. (1984:6)

Whether the approach is bio-medical or socio-relational, it usually features the same discourse sequence composed of three parts: asking questions, answering, and expressing an acknowledgement – and sometimes providing an assessment of the last statement that was made by the patient (Coupland et al. 1994; Fisher & Groce 1990; Pauwels 1995). However, some specific differences occur depending on which approach the doctor uses throughout the consultation. Whereas the bio-medical approach tends to favour a discourse directed towards the body part in need of restoration or cure, isolating the sickness from the whole person, the socio-relational approach aims to focus on the patient as a whole, as a person who lives their life as part of a social network who is currently suffering from a medical condition.

For Mishler, the medical discourse is divided into two distinct and antagonistic voices: the "voice of the lifeworld" disrupts and interrupts the dominant "voice of medicine" (1984:63). This view has been criticized by Barry et al. (2001) who claim that doctors modulate their speech depending on whether they perceive their patients to be complaining from physical or psychological problems. Silverman (1987) perceives medical discourse as an interactional speech activity that allows the socio-relational frame to interact at any time with the bio-medical one. His idea of the interaction of voices is also expressed by Cohen-Cole (1991), who developed, in conjunction with Julian Bird, a three-function approach to the medical interview that responds to the medical condition of patients as well as their emotional and motivational needs. The three functions consist of:

a. Gathering data to understand the patient's problem.
b. Developing rapport and responding to the patient's emotions.
c. Fostering patient education and motivation.

The incorporation of these three functions into the medical consultation creates a framework for doctors to gather accurate information about their patient's health, to educate the patient in relation to the prescribed treatment, and to explore emotional and social issues that may influence the health outcome. Thus, the

> Three-function model of the interview represents an operationalized application of the biopsychosocial model designed to facilitate doctor–patient communication processes. (Cohen-Cole 1991:7)

(The bio-psycho-social model stresses that both psychological and social variables play a crucial role in the development, course and outcome of all illnesses. See Cohen-Cole 1991, 1994; Engel 1974.) The three-function model of communication, therefore, understands the medical consultation as an opportunity to care for the whole person of the patient by amalgamating the *voice of the lifeworld* with the *voice of medicine*. Against this, Todd and Fisher (1993) in their studies of medical discourse argue that doctors and patients understand the exchange in a different way. They found that doctors mainly operate in the bio-medical frame, while patients bring the socio-relational frame to the discourse.

2.6 Doctor–patient communication: The medical and linguistic perspectives

The investigation of doctor–patient communication has generally been undertaken within two major traditions. Studies conducted by medical researchers establish themselves within a sociological framework (Cohen-Cole 1991; Neighbour 1987); these emphasize the ways in which communication can promote patient satisfaction (Burgoon et al. 1991; Roter et al. 1987) and lead ultimately to the patient's recovery. The linguistic (or micro-analytical) tradition, on the other hand, emphasizes the communication strategies used in the doctor–patient interview and the variables (sex, age, social status, etc.) that influence the development of the discourse (Blanchard et al. 1988; Charon et al. 1994; Fisher 1995; Fisher & Todd 1986; Irish & Hall 1995; Sundquist 1995). Here I review both traditions, arguing with Charon et al. that analytical and micro-analytical analyses of doctor–patient interactions complement each other, and that a synthetic approach is likely to shed the most light on the subject. The following section explores the medical approaches to doctor–patient communication; this will be followed by an overview of the research carried out by linguists in the field.

2.6.1 Medical approaches to doctor–patient communication

Early attempts at establishing a framework for the study of doctor–patient communication emphasized structural and semantic aspects of discourse (Cassell et al. 1976). Subsequent research focused on the dominant role of the doctor in the interview (Epstein et al. 1993; von Raffler-Engel 1989). More recently, a paradigm shift has seen the incorporation of the patient's perspective into a relationship-centred medical model of communication (Drew 2001; Roter 2000; Stivers & Heritage 2001; Thompson 1998). Much work still needs to be done, however, since variables such as gender remain under-researched (Gabbardalley 1995).

In a comprehensive review, Ong et al. (1995) identified three main aims of doctor–patient communication:

a. To create a good inter-personal relationship.
b. To exchange information.
c. To make treatment-related decisions.

Doctors can create good inter-personal relationships with their patients by incorporating a lifeworld approach (Mishler 1984), and by adopting empathic techniques such as establishing eye contact, eliciting feelings, paraphrasing and reflecting, using silence and non-verbal communication, listening to what the patient is saying (and to what s/he is unable to say), making encouraging replies, and including semi-verbal, non-specific utterances such as "hm-hm, ah" (Bensing 1991; Ong et al. 1995). In a study of the communication styles used by doctors in an oncology consultation, Dowsett et al. (2000) found that individuals watching a videotape of the event significantly preferred a patient-centred approach to a bio-medical one. Establishing an environment conducive to good inter-personal relationships can be jeopardized by the doctor's refusal or inability to engage the empathic techniques listed above.

The exchange of information is a two-way process: information is both sought and given. Doctors need to obtain information from their patients in order to make a diagnosis, and patients must describe their symptoms in a way that is understandable to their doctors. Thus, although the relationship between doctor and patient has been depicted traditionally as a paternalistic one, with many patients still thinking that "the doctor should take primary responsibility in the decision-making process" (Ong et al. 1995: 905), the process has to be understood as one of mutual obligation and responsibility if there is to be a positive outcome. Patients need cure and care in their treatment, where cure depends on knowing and understanding, and care relates to the feeling of being known and understood (Ong et al. 1995).

Doctors sometimes underestimate the patient's desire for information (Ong et al. 1995). This is currently being emphasized in *emancipatory models*, where appreciation of patient expertise is recognized as being at the core of good doctor–patient communication (Thorne et al. 2000). Historically, patient participation in the consultation has not always been satisfactorily achieved. Heath (1992) analysed video recordings of doctor–patient interviews in the UK in order to investigate how patients receive a doctor's diagnosis. He found that the manner in which the doctor delivered the diagnosis could silence the patient. Even when the doctor left a pause after making the announcement, the patient sometimes still felt uneasy and unable to ask questions or voice concerns, particularly if the doctor was preoccupied with another task, such as writing out a prescription. At such times, patients may believe that talk would be inappropriate, and limit their utterances to a downward-intoned "er" or "yeh".

While Heath (1992) found that patient participation increased when there was a mismatch between the diagnosis and the patient's lay knowledge of the medical condition, since this prompted the patient to seek clarification, the opposite can also be true: the doctor's use of technical terms that have a different lay meaning can cause frustration and confusion to the patient, leading to a lack of compliance (Daly & Hulka 1975; Hadlow & Pitts 1991). Patients appear to be sensitive not only to their differential knowledge of the medical lexicon, but also to the amount of information provided to them. Hahn (1995: 168) observes that

> Patients who receive more information are much more likely to be satisfied with the encounter, much more likely to understand and recall the information received, and more likely to comply with the physician's recommendation.

While the amount of information provided by doctors may be dependent on the individual patient's desire for it, patient satisfaction is achieved, *inter alia*, if doctors are not dominant and their style not controlling (Ong et al. 1995). Ong et al. also found that there is a correlation between good communication and patient satisfaction, compliance, recall and understanding of medical information. Overall, patient *dis*satisfaction has been shown to be related to:

a. The absence of warmth and friendliness on the part of the doctor.
b. A failure to fulfil patient expectations.
c. The use of confusing terminology and instructions.

Charles et al. (1997) propose a model of *shared decision-making* in the medical encounter, which they structure as four main building-blocks:

a. Both patient and doctor are involved in the consultation.
b. Both parties share information.
c. Both build a consensus about the preferred treatment.
d. Both reach an agreement on the treatment to be implemented.

However, Stevenson et al. (2000) studied 62 consultations between patients and general practitioners and found little evidence of this model of *shared decision-making* in practice. In their study, some of the consultations did not even present the last two (c and d) of the four conditions suggested by Charles et al.: that is, they did not achieve doctor–patient consensus on the medical treatment to be followed, nor on the way it would be accomplished. In spite of this finding, there is a sound recognition – in research studies, at least – of the need for doctors and patients to reach a mutual agreement that takes into consideration their respective knowledge and wishes. Happily, Bissell et al. (2003), following the recommendations of a multi-disciplinary group of health providers based in the UK (Working Party 1997), found a new tendency to manage doctor–patient communication based on partnership and collaboration.

Thus far we have shown that at the core of a successful medical consultation is patient satisfaction leading to proper compliance with medical recommendations (see Burgoon et al. 1991; Gerber 1986; Korsch et al. 1968; Lebarère 2003; Lieberman 1996; Roter et al. 1987; Stearns & Ross 1993; Williams et al. 1998); and patient satisfaction, in turn, is due in large part to good doctor–patient communication. Compliance, therefore, as Daly and Hulka (1975) concluded after analysing questionnaires and interviewing patients, results from a good relationship with the doctor. For example, in a study carried out in an epilepsy clinic in South India, Gopinath et al. (2000) found that there was a significant positive correlation between effective doctor–patient communication and compliance. In sum, good communication, as part of a patient-centred approach, is the key to compliance and effective health management (Bensing 1991).

It is interesting to note however that the concept of compliance has not escaped controversy (Bissell et al. 2003; Kreps 1988; Thompson 1998; Walker et al. 2002). A patient may be "compliant" in the sense of following medical instructions without participating in the decision-making process. Indeed, it must be allowed that some (though not most) patients even prefer their doctors to behave in an aloof and authoritarian manner. Accordingly, Bissell et al.

use the term *concordance* to indicate the equal participation of doctor and patient in the consultation with the aim of achieving a *therapeutic coalition*. In this present study, compliance and adherence will be used as synonyms to indicate simply that the patient has followed a medical recommendation. Any extra information about the roles of participants in the event will be provided when appropriate.

Donovan and Blake (1992) found that between one-third and one-half of all patients in their study were non-compliant, although the reasons for this varied. Non-complying patients tended to carry out a *cost-benefit* analysis of each treatment, with their perceptions and social circumstances at the core of their decision-making. This means that an apparently irrational act of non-compliance, from the doctor's perspective, may be a completely rational act as far as the patient is concerned. Lebarère et al. (2003), in their study carried out in France, aimed at understanding whether patients who had consulted the telephone medical line had complied with the recommendation given to them 48 hours previously. Results showed a staggering compliance rate of over 80 percent. In this instance, compliance appeared to correlate to patient expectations, the perceived appropriateness of the recommendation, and patient satisfaction.

Hitherto the discussion has been on doctor–patient communication from the point of view of research carried out mainly in the fields of social science and medicine. These studies, however, tend to gloss over issues of discourse in the relationship. The following two sections present an overview of the linguistic approaches to medical discourse, from both the doctor's and then the patient's perspective.

2.6.2 Linguistic approaches: The doctor's perspective

A number of studies carried out in the area of doctor–patient communication have focused on the miscommunication that occurs in the clinical setting. Problems of communication appear to increase when two different languages and/or cultural groups interact, as in the case of Hispanics, mainly from Central America, living in the United States and interacting with Anglo-American doctors (Erzinger 1989; Kline & Acosta 1980; Muñoz 1981; Prince 1986). However, miscommunication does not necessarily disappear when the participants are from the same cultural group and speak the same language (Bamberg 1991; Byrne & Long 1976; Thompson & Pledger 1993).

Byrne and Long have pioneered research in the area of doctor–patient communication with their analysis of 2,000 visits to general practitioners in Great

Britain, focusing on the interaction that emerged during the diagnostic stage. They observed that doctors controlled the exchange and that the contribution of patients was restricted mainly to the end of the consultation. Shuy (1983) describes the control exercised by doctors as most apparent in the preference they show for asking questions, introducing topics and shunning a balanced participation. Bias in the use of questions is also evident in Coulthard and Ashby's early studies (1975) and in Ong et al.'s (1995) review.

Frankel (1984, 1990) and Ten Have (1991) note that questions have been a major topic of study, and the large number of works published in this area confirm their observation (Coulthard & Ashby 1975, 1976; Kess 1984; Mulholland 1994; Rozholdova 1999; Seijo et al. 1991; West 1984, 1990). Their function is usually medically oriented, tending to centre on the onset and development of the condition up to the time of presentation, or on the patient's progress since the previous visit. Doctors' questions have been studied with a view to:

a. Observing their linguistic form.
b. Assessing their relative use by both participants.
c. Investigating and categorizing their functions in a medical interaction.
d. Observing sequences of usage.
e. Investigating the social variables that may lead doctors to modify their speech.

Coulthard and Ashby (1975) enumerate three kinds of questions used by doctors:

a. Testing exchanges, where the information is transferred in the next move, which may be identified by particular responses (e.g. "good", "that's right") or by a high-key "yes".
b. Transfer exchanges, where the doctor uses "yes" or repeats what the patient has said.
c. Matching exchanges, where the first speaker presents something to be confirmed, and the second confirms it.

These authors show that the doctor takes control of the interview by asking questions aimed at getting information about the patient's health, while often disregarding additional information the patient may provide. Jones (2001) also found that doctors often did not respond to additional "newsworthy" material the patient appended to their answers. West (1984) notes that doctors initiate the majority of questions and that the kinds of question they ask in the consultation influence the patient's contributions. Questions made in sequence and multiple-choice questions do not inspire much of an answer from patients because of "constraining structural circumstances" (West 1984:82). The way in which the question is presented, therefore, can pre-determine the reply.

As far as questioning sequences are concerned, Coupland et al. (1994) observe that these often take the form of a three-part structure. The doctor initiates the topic, the patient responds to it, and the doctor retakes the floor to express a third-position assessment. Other studies have observed how the function attached to questions can modulate a patient's contribution. Royster (1990) found that some questions were intended to elicit a patient's knowledge and understanding of his/her health condition. She called these *probing questions*. Similarly, Fisher (1993:170) observed that some questioning strategies offer the opportunity to patients to show their competence in medical discourse.

However, questions are not the exclusive discourse form used by doctors to gain information. Bergmann (1992) studied the interaction between psychiatrists and their patients, and found that specialists do not always use direct questions; they may simply use an assertion as a way of making the patient volunteer information. This technique has been called *fishing* by Pomerantz (1992). For Bergmann, it is a recurrent feature of his data.

Questions and interruptions by doctors have been interpreted as a form of control (Ong et al. 1995) exercised over the patient. Buller and Buller (1987) identify two kinds of behaviour manifested by doctors – affiliation and control. Control is expressed through domination of the conversation, verbal exaggeration (to emphasize a point) and dramatization (being very argumentative, and constantly making gestures when communicating). Control may also manifest itself in the tendency of some doctors to interrupt their patients' discourse with questions (Irish & Hall 1995). On the whole, however, the use of questions by doctors seems to be much more complex and varied. Harres (1996, 1998) analysed 29 audio-taped consultations and found that "tag questions" were used by doctors not only as control mechanisms but also as involvement strategies. Doctors used tag questions (such as "But basically you're feeling well, are you?") to:

a. Elicit information from patients.
b. Summarize and confirm information.
c. Express empathy.
d. Give positive feedback.

Mulholland (1994) believes it is important to distinguish between directives and *multiple directives* in the consultative exchange: that is, the doctor's single utterances which include more than one command. Multiple directives can be identified as a coherent unit in the speech, requiring the patient to engage in a "single complex task, a single set of related tasks, or a set of tasks which, from the speaker's point of view, have a single goal" (1994:75). As such, Mulholland understands the exchange between doctor and patient as an interactional phenomenon, in contrast to West's view of the consultation as one defined by independent directives. Mulholland also draws attention to the greater potential for misunderstanding and confusion, and hence for non-compliance, when multiple directives are given to the patient.

As for studies on the discourse strategies used to bring about a less asymmetrical interaction, the work of Ten Have (1991) in Holland is worth mentioning. Contrary to the description above of three-part discourse sequences, Ten Have observed, using a critical analysis framework, that doctors sometimes used the particle "oh" at the beginning of their third turn in such a way that it was not intended to express an assessment of the patient's last utterance(s). Atkinson (1992) found that third turns, such as "mhm O.K." and "mhm, ah", as studied by Bensing (1991), showed a similar tendency. Coupland et al. also recorded a third-position lexicon item in their data. For them,

> The term "continuer" is most appropriately applied to non-referring expressions (such as *uh-huh* or *yes*) uttered with high-rise contours, or to referring expressions which request patients to elaborate upon a summary account (such as *Not well?*), said with a fall-rise on the tonic syllable. (1994:117)

Importantly, Coupland et al. suggest that while a third-position continuer can encourage the patient to continue the narrative, it can also inhibit further speech if it is uttered with a low-falling contour.

Finally, while Bensing (1991) observed that eye contact with patients helped to create rapport, Ong et al. (1995) found that doctors' touching and proximity were considered breaches of patient privacy, a view shared by Parrott et al. (1989) and Parrott (1994). Interestingly, this attitude was not shared by Chilean patients in Scarpaci's (1988) study, since Chileans did not feel that their territorial space was threatened when their doctor came close to them. Scarpaci's study was carried out in a Villa O'Higgins clinic and aimed at understanding the satisfaction rate of 140 frequent users of the National Health Service System (SNS). The clinic was located in an area where "most low-income residents live" (Scarpaci 1988:200), and it was found that:

> Physicians who listen to, examine, and touch patients provide support in the difficult and stressful lives of the urban poor. (1988:208)

2.6.3 Linguistic approaches: The patient's perspective

While doctors perceive the medical exchange primarily as an encounter within bio-medical and socio-relational frames, patients tend to present their health problem as a personal condition, with associated socio-cultural and psychological implications (Andary et al. 2003; Helman 1994; Mishler 1984). These different views of illness may influence whether the medical consultation takes place at all. Defining oneself as ill usually involves both an objective and a subjective experience, which might include changes in body appearance, regular bodily functions and bodily emissions; changes in motor ability and emotional state; behavioural changes towards others as well as changes in any of the five major senses; the experience of unusual physical discomfort (Helman 1994: 109). However, in anthropological medicine it has been shown that patients belonging to different cultural groups generally declare themselves ill when:

> There is an agreement between [their] perception of impaired well-being, and the perception of those around [them]. (Helman 1994: 110)

The realization that a health provider's help is needed is the first step towards making the medical visit possible.

According to Helman, illness is interpreted as a socio-cultural process that involves both the person who is sick, because s/he is experiencing something unusual in him/herself, and those around the person who is unwell, who detect changes in the individual's state and comment on them. It has been reported that Mexican-American children interpret the *hearing of voices* as a religious experience, whereas Anglo-American teenagers interpret the same phenomenon as a sign of insanity or hallucination (Quesada 1976). In this case, Mexican-Americans may not see the need to seek medical help as would their Anglo-American counterparts. Similarly, some illnesses may not be viewed as requiring medical intervention because of a cultural belief that differs from medical practice. Quesada (1976) has shown how the *cosmology of destiny* – with its implications for illness and death – can be a factor in determining whether a Mexican-American visits a doctor. While some complaints are perceived as detrimental to good health and therefore need medical treatment, others are not considered life-threatening since "nobody has died from [them]". Here the macro representation of socio-cultural realities (the cosmology of destiny) is applied to in order to interpret the micro reality of the unwell individual.

Even when the visit does take place, problems may still arise. It has been shown by Rehbein (1994) that when participants do not share the same concept of illness, a schema conflict (Tannen & Wallat 1993) is likely to occur. This was the case in a consultation reported by Rehbein (1994), in which a Spanish-speaking patient interacting with a German doctor led to a mismatch in the concepts of obesity and mental illness. The patient interpreted obesity as a hereditary condition and mental illness as a synonym for being crazy, whereas the doctor assessed both of these problems as two medical illnesses requiring treatment. Kleinman (1980) comments that illness is usually described within an "explanatory model" that accounts for the origin and time of occurrence of the condition, its cause, severity, and the relevant treatment. Different categories of people (lay, medical), however, may use different explanatory models.

As another example of a mismatched conception of illness, I recall an example given by Andary et al. (2003). Danny was a 22 year-old Australian male of Lebanese parents. The Western doctor interpreted Danny's distant and non-engaging behaviour with his family as a reaction against Lebanese traditional cultural values, instead of recognizing it as a call for psychiatric care. Andary et al. summarized the situation thus:

> The client and the mental health professional have brought to the clinical interaction different cultural values, different assumptions about the expression and meaning of distress and differences in their beliefs, "explanatory models", and treatment expectations. (2003: 10)

Doctor–patient communication may depend therefore on the extent to which the doctor is able to identify the patient's own socio-cultural framework for illness and negotiate appropriate treatment without provoking a schema conflict.

Let us now examine the ways in which patient participation affects the exchange. The achievement of communicative competence on the part of the patient is sometimes no easy task. Lacoste (1981) analysed the different strategies used by patients to make their needs known to their doctors, despite the obvious asymmetry in knowledge that existed between them. She describes instances of "territorial disputes", as in the case of a patient who used an inappropriate, non-technical word to describe his symptoms. This created tension and served as a sharp reminder that patients should stay in their own territory. When a patient takes the initiative, the doctor may indicate displeasure with such strategies as silence, not terminating a response, announcing but not giving a response, taking another initiative (e.g. asking a question) or giving a purely formal acknowledgement. The patient may also use *dramatization* in order to achieve what s/he desires, playing with the doctor through such specific discursive strategies as mocking and self-irony (Grainger 2002; Lacoste 1981).

Irish and Hall (1995) studied video-taped doctor–patient consultations for interruptive and overlapping speech by both participants. They found that patients engaged in significantly more of this speech behaviour than doctors, and that they interrupted more with statements, whereas doctors tended to interrupt with questions.

In an experimental study, McCann and Weinman (1996) provided a group of patients with an intervention leaflet that encouraged them to take an active role in the consultation; a control group was simply given a leaflet containing dietary advice. The results showed that patients in the intervention group had significantly longer consultations than those in the control group and that they asked more questions. Although there was no significant change in the intervention patients' level of satisfaction, it is interesting to note that the doctors tended to feel that they had a better understanding of these patients because more information was exchanged. This empirical finding suggests the importance of dialogue during the consultation because, although patient satisfaction was not at issue, the information gained by doctors may have helped them to give a better diagnosis and propose a more appropriate treatment.

An improved doctor–patient relationship may lead to the patient's greater competence and well-being. Therapeutic results are likely to be better for competent patients (see Gruninger 1995 for a review). In spite of this, Gopinath et al. (2000) concluded that one-third of the patients in their study received insufficient information about epilepsy and its treatment from the doctor. In another study, Blanchard et al. (1988) found that a majority of cancer patients wanted to be wholly informed, no matter how positive or negative the information was. However, older patients were more likely than younger ones to follow an authoritarian model during the consultation by decreasing their level of participation.

The failure of doctors to acknowledge the patient's own expertise has been shown to lead to a spiral of mutual alienation in cases of chronic disease (Thorne et al. 2000). The patient's participation in the medical discourse depends to a large extent on the opportunities given and on the appropriateness of the linguistic features and strategies used by doctors in the institutional setting. At the same time, Heath (1992) points out that the patient's reluctance to engage in the discourse creates and maintains the asymmetry throughout the exchange.

West, in her investigation of question sequences used in the medical consultation, found that, of a total of 773 questions, only 9% were initiated by patients and 91% by doctors. Of interest is her comment that "given their scarcity, it is notable that patient-initiated questions failed to elicit answers from physicians more often than the reverse" (1984: 84). She notes that the stammered questions of some patients may have been the reason for the doctor's lack of response. Korsch et al. (1968) corroborate the view that patients' questions are frequently disregarded by doctors. West (1984) also explores the possibility that questions may be interpreted as an intrusion into medical territory and as a threat to the doctor's status and authority.

The discourse style of patients in their responses to doctors can also influence the consultation. Coupland et al. (1994) observed that patients very rarely responded to the initial question "How are you?" with a medically oriented answer. Instead, they interpreted the question as a request to initiate the talk. Of the 80 initial questions reported in Coupland et al.'s study, 54 received an answer that was related to the patient's lifeworld. Nonetheless, the simple fact of listening to patients recounting their stories is considered by Coupland et al. as a valuable starting-point in the medical consultation. Davis (1988: 230) observes that this is made possible when both doctor and patient work together in the exchange:

> Recounting the trouble, like getting the floor is an interactional accomplishment, requiring specific tasks from both the patient as a trouble-teller and from the GP as a trouble-recipient.

Despite this, Mishler (1984) notes that doctors often ignore and disregard the personal experiences of patients, favouring those contributions that are medically oriented or those that give factually based answers to medical issues. To summarize:

a. The patient's discourse style can have an effect on the interaction.
b. Territorial disputes are likely to occur if the patient takes the initiative in the medical discourse.
c. The patient's preferred treatment and management will depend on the individual and on the kind of illness s/he is suffering from.
d. Patients may increase their participation in the speech if doctors use linguistic strategies that favour their contribution.

The outcome of the consultation, like any other speech encounter, is also dependent on a number of sociological factors, including the socio-economic class, education and gender of the participants. The following section reviews some of the most prominent studies in this area.

2.7 Sociological factors and doctor–patient communication

While there is a flourishing literature that explores gender difference as a variable in patients' interaction with doctors (Ainsworth-Vaughn 1994, 1998; Atkinson 1992; Borges 1986; Coupland et al. 1994; Davis 1988; Dawson et al. 2000; Fisher 1995; Harres 1996, 1998; Heath 1992; Hein & Wodak 1987; Maynard 1992; Pauwels 1995; Todd 1993; Todd & Fisher 1993; West 1984, 1990; Wodak 1996), relatively few studies have analysed the ways in which a patient's age, social class or education influence the exchange.

In Western societies, the medical profession has usually been associated with high social prestige and high annual income:

> The medical profession can be seen as a healing "sub-culture", with its own world view. In the process of medical education the students ... also acquire a high social status, high earning power and socially legitimated role of healer which carries with it certain rights and obligations. (Helman 1994: 101)

The social class and education of the patient, on the other hand, cannot be predicted in the same way. As we reminded ourselves in the introduction, we are all potential patients. However, it is worth noting that causes of illness in anthropological medicine are closely linked to social factors (Helman 1994) and that patients from lower social classes have been shown to be more likely to suffer particular kinds of illnesses (Navarro 1990; Pollard & Hyatt 1999; Sundquist 1995). Further, being a member of a lower socio-economic class is often an indicator of poor health (Blaxter 1987; Navarro 1990). Taking a cross-cultural perspective, Pollard and Hyatt (1999) report the high incidence of fatal infections, accidents, poisoning and violence in both females and males in Guatemala, in contrast to the USA, where those causes of death were relatively under-represented, and where ischaemic heart disease claimed the most lives.

Age, social class and education appear to be variables that affect communication between doctor and patient. Roter and Hall (1992) quote previous studies carried out in both the USA and UK showing an upward correlation between the patient's social class and the doctor's level of engagement. Waitzkin (1985) found that patients of higher social class and better educational background spent more time in the consultation and received a larger quantity of information. It has also been shown that educated people tend to challenge the doctor's authority more often (White et al. 1984). White et al. also found that younger patients were more likely to confront their doctors than older ones.

As regards gender health in the West, studies on the degree of interaction of female patients in the consultation have yielded contrasting results. Although some women feel that asking questions is considered inappropriate behaviour (McKenzie 2002), other studies indicate that it is precisely the greater number of questions that women ask that allows physicians to give more information to females than to males (Pendleton & Bochner 1980; Roter & Hall 1992; Waitzkin 1985; Wallen et al. 1979). Roter and Hall's study, based on 100 routine medical visits to a teaching hospital, found that physicians used more medical jargon with their female patients, which prompted the women to ask more questions to clarify those terms. Roter and Hall (1992:43) indicate that

> Female patients also gave more information of a medical nature to the doctor than male patients did – perhaps in reciprocation of receiving more technical language.

These social factors may have an effect not only on the development of the discourse but also on subsequent medical management. For example, Fisher found that young white females were more likely to be managed conservatively and older Mexican-American women more likely to be given a hysterectomy when both groups presented with the same health problem (1993:166). Littlewood (1999) found a tendency to prescribe more tranquillizers to females than to males to overcome psychological distress.

Linguistic studies of doctor–patient communication, therefore, need to take into account the complex socio-cultural and socio-economic variables interacting in the exchange. In the present study an attempt has been made to keep the social class and cultural group of participants as similar as possible, while the distribution of patients' ages has been controlled. For reasons outlined in the next chapter, gender-based differences will be studied to a limited extent only.

2.8 Conclusion

A review of the literature on doctor–patient communication from a variety of disciplines has indicated the desirability of medical consultations in which both doctor and patient play a participatory role. Non-linguistic approaches may give us much important information about the consultation process, but they leave unexamined the development of the discourse and thus limit their chances of detecting, understanding and solving any overall failure in communication. Discourse analytical tools allow us to better recognize problems of communication by focusing on the dynamics of the verbal exchange. I shall show in this work that a more favourable outcome for both doctor and patient can be achieved when recommendations for particular communicative strategies, based on the findings of critical discourse analysis, are implemented in medical consultations.

Note

1. This passage has also been chosen by Schiffrin (1994:7) for her discussion on interactional socio-linguistics.

Chapter 3

Doctor–patient communication

An empirical study

While some studies of doctor–patient communication have been developed within a narrowly defined framework of discourse analysis, others have adopted a more eclectic approach. As Cameron observes, this points to "the interdisciplinary nature of discourse analysis" (2001:47).

Conversation analysis (CA) has a long history in the study of medical discourse in its application to systematic attempts at discovering sequencing and orderedness in doctor–patient interactions (Beach 2001; Sarangi 2001; Stivers & Heritage 2001; Ten Have 1991, to mention a few). Although deeply rooted in the ethnomethodological tradition, the key point of this approach, following the school of thought founded by Garfinkel, is to observe how certain conversational rules are followed in the interaction and how these tend to promote order in the exchange of discourse sequences. The limitations of CA for the present study are that it operates only at the micro level and does not offer a way of linking the data of individual conversations to the broader sociological frame.

The *Pragmatics* tradition originates from the philosophy of language of Austin (1962), Grice (1971) and Searle (1969). It attempts to comprehend how language is used in context, and the meaning that the speaker and hearer may give to a particular utterance. In the area of doctor–patient communication attention has been given to the *model of politeness* developed by Brown and Levinson (1987) and the conceptualization of *face* as posited by Goffman (1967). Some of the studies in this area have researched nurse–patient discourse (Spiers 1998), paediatric discourse (looking at the three-party exchange of doctor–parent–child) (Aronsson & Rundström 1989), verbal play in hospital wards (Grainger 2002), and the effect on *face* of non-compliant patients visiting a medical practitioner (Cordella in press).

An influential approach that aims at detecting how the discourse may reveal unbalanced social relationships and inequities in an institutional setting is *Critical discourse analysis*, rooted in both structural linguistics and critical theory (see Cameron 2001 for an overview of critical theory and spoken discourse approaches). The nexus between language and society and society and language is reflected in the dialectic relationship of the discourse: speakers reproduce ideas embedded in their societal group and by so doing tend to perpetuate those ideas within society (Fairclough 1985, 1992, 1995; van Dijk 1995a, 1996, 1997b; Wodak 1989, 1996, 1999a). Hein and Wodak (1987) and Labov and Fanshel (1977) have explored medical discourse from this perspective and have also incorporated pragmatics into their analysis.

3.1 Discourse analysis: Interactional socio-linguistics and ethnographic approaches

The choice of methodology for the analysis of the medical consultations set out below was bound to the research questions that this study aims to answer. Both *interactional socio-linguistics* and *ethnographic* approaches to discourse analysis have been favoured, since these complement each other in their understanding of discourse as a socio-cultural event. Following van Dijk (1987: 32–33):

> Discourse [is] a form of social interaction between social members taking place in social contexts that are constrained by (interpreted) social structures and cultural frameworks.

Discourse analysis provides the theoretical basis and the analytical tools necessary to understand which forms of talk doctors and patients use in the consultation and can be used to interpret what is taking place around these forms of talk. By using an interactional socio-linguistics approach to discourse analysis, the speech of participants can be divided into small units or episodes (van Dijk 1982) that share descriptive similarities, such as questioning, story-telling, or affiliative discourse strategies. In addition, the interactional socio-linguistic approach aids in the interpretation of the speech by both providing an account of the individual discourse and connecting it to the broader institutional and socio-cultural frame. These findings in combination may then reveal a situation that favours good communication or one that hampers it by creating "disorders in discourse" (Wodak 1996).

The ethnographic approach analyses the spoken interaction (e.g. doctor–patient communication) in association with a particular social setting (e.g. the Clinic) and "studies patterns of observed and recorded communicative behaviour" (Stubbs 1983: 40). Accordingly, this study is based on observed, recorded information and tape-recorded naturalistic data.

While Chapter 6 (*The Fellow Human voice*) uses conversation analysis tools to record a localized event, interpretation of the data requires external socio-cultural knowledge in order to build up a comprehensive understanding of the interaction. It has therefore been necessary to incorporate different approaches to achieve the aims of this study. My objective is to provide, whenever possible, an interpretation of the micro production of the discourse while also accounting for the macro context as defined by socio-cultural practices.

3.2 Research design

In what follows I outline the research design implemented in this study, and give an overview of the medical institution, doctors and patients involved in the research. The specific aspects of the discourse that became the focus of my analysis were selected following a "bottom-up" approach. Once the transcriptions of doctor–patient conversations were completed, the linguistic behaviour of the participants was surveyed in order to determine whether there were any obvious general trends. In the process of familiarization with the data it emerged that both the doctor and the patient were performing different forms of talk during the medical interview. As a result, I carried out a formal analysis to distinguish between these forms of talk and to provide a way of understanding the interaction that occurred. The analysis concentrates on the talk that forms part of the two communication routines of the medical consultation classified by Pauwels (1995) as *History-taking* and *Management and treatment of a health problem or health issue*. Pauwels's framework is discussed further below.

These communication routines are of great interest especially in the context of follow-up visits, since the doctor and patient will already have met at least once before. Whereas the initial visit will usually involve the doctor informing the patient of a provisional diagnosis, educating the patient about the medical problem, proposing or advising and explaining a therapy or a physical or manipulative procedure, providing reassurance and arranging a follow-up visit or referral, follow-up visits differ in that diagnoses have already been discussed with the patient, and the emphasis is on the assessment of test results and the patient's ongoing management. The doctor will probably check on previous details and introduce new material to the talk. Follow-up visits constitute a rich source of information for analysis, since they involve monitoring of the patient's progress and compliance; and because patients generally have a better understanding of their condition, they may have prepared a number of questions they wish to raise with their doctor.

The research questions that are the focus of this study are followed by an overview of the health system in Chile and a description of the main characteristics of the Clinic where this project took place. There follows a description of the medical consulting rooms and the equipment used for the recording of the data. Data was collected between September and December 1997 and is presented in four stages: Stage I: observation period; Stage II: questionnaire; Stage III: semi-structured interview; Stage IV: tape-recording of the medical consultation. Participants involved in each of these stages are also profiled, noting the selection criteria used in the process. A description of how the analysis was carried out and the limitations that such an analysis might have are also provided. The final part of the chapter explores the ethical issues and permits involved in the study.

3.3 Research questions

The main aim of the present study is to expand our current knowledge of medical discourse through an investigation of doctor–patient communication in a Chilean clinic. Specifically, in this research I intend to:

1. Investigate Chilean doctor–patient communication and discover the forms of talk that participants use in consultations.
2. Describe the interaction between doctors' and patients' forms of talk in the consultation.
3. Explore the role of power and affiliative discourse in the consultation.
4. Investigate whether the participation framework of the consultation presents a dynamic interaction.
5. Explore whether there is a connection between the discourse at the micro level of the consultation and broader socio-cultural practices operating at the macro level of society.

3.4 The Chilean health care system

At the time of data collection for this research the health care system in Chile offered two major health care plans: a public one and a private one. Chileans could "choose" either of the two, although the choice was generally determined

Table 1. Distribution of health insurance cover in the Chilean population

Health cover system	Population in thousands	%
FONASA (Public health system)	8,809	68.8%
ISAPRES (Private health system)	1,927	15.1%
FF.AA. (Army health system)	318	2.5%
Particulares (Full fee paying)	1,550	12.1%
Other (Other medical plans)	197	1.5%
TOTAL	12,801	100%

(Data from Giaconi 1994)

by the monthly family income. According to Giaconi (1994), 68.8% of the population have public health cover (FONASA), whereas only 15.1% have private cover (ISAPRE). A total of 2.5% of the population have health cover provided by the Armed Forces (FFAA), and 12.1% are *particulares* who pay a full fee when visiting a doctor since they have no particular health cover. The remaining 1.5% have medical cover which has not yet been classified (see Table 1).

Chileans with public health cover may attend health clinics (*policlínicos*) run by the *Sistema Nacional de Servicio de Salud* (SNSS), or visit outpatient clinics run by the *Fondo Nacional de Salud* (FONASA). Under the current system, fees are determined by the patient's monthly income and the medical specialist being consulted (cardiology, oncology, radiology, etc.). León (2000) provides a review of the Chilean national health system and an introduction to historical developments between 1983 and 2000.

3.5 The research site: The PUC Outpatient Clinic

Doctor–patient communication has been widely studied in different specific settings and some patterns of linguistic behaviour appear to be sensitive to the environmental context. For example, the talk in an emergency department will probably be different from that of a follow-up consultation. Accordingly, it is important that the location and context of the research investigation be made explicit and described in detail.

At the time of this research the Pontificia Universidad Católica de Chile (PUC) in Santiago had a medical network made up of four *Centros asistenciales* (Medical Clinics). The first of these, the PUC hospital itself, is located in the city centre, and has a casualty department and an oupatient and inpatient teaching hospital. The three remaining centres are positioned strategically around the metropolitan area of Santiago (in the suburbs of San Joaquín, Irarrázaval and Las Condes). Patients are free to visit the centre closest to them. The data for this study was collected in the Outpatient Clinic of the PUC located in San Joaquín, a working-class suburb in the south-east part of Santiago.

The census held in 1992 (*Instituto Nacional de Estadísticas, Chile*, 1992) recorded the population of San Joaquín as 114,017 inhabitants, representing 2.16% of the total population of the metropolitan area. The average monthly salary of those people living in the suburb who visited the Clinic was in the range of Aust$750.[1]

The San Joaquín Clinic used in this study is a teaching centre that trains both medical students and *internistas* (medical graduates). Junior health professionals are supervised by a group of experienced doctors whose responsibility it is to ensure that the diagnosis and treatment given to patients are correct. This particular Clinic is one of the few innovative tertiary institutions in Chile interested in research on doctor–patient communication: a subject on the topic is offered to students in the final years of their course. The Clinic also encourages patients to be aware of doctor–patient communication issues by suggesting they assess trainee doctors; it invites scholars to talk on this topic and fosters postgraduate research on patient satisfaction. In addition, the PUC runs health awareness and disease prevention campaigns and public lectures throughout the year as part of its education programme.

The Clinic had, at the time of this research, 39 medical areas divided into specific departments – Cardiology, Endocrinology, Gerontology, Pathology, General Medicine, Oncology, Psychiatry, and so on – and laboratory areas for blood tests and X-rays. On-site laboratory facilities allow patients to consult a doctor and have any prescribed tests performed in the same Centre. The San Joaquín Clinic is not used exclusively by local residents; it also attracts middle-class patients who come from a number of suburbs in Santiago or from the provinces.[2] The number of female patients is almost double that of males, according to statistics collected by the Centre.

3.5.1 The consultation room at PUC

Upon arrival at the Clinic, patients take a seat in one of the two waiting rooms used for general medicine. One is in an area where there are three consulting rooms and a staff room, and the other is in an area where there are four consulting rooms and an Information Desk. A corridor separates the two waiting rooms. The consulting rooms have aluminium walls, glass windows and two doors, one of which connects to the patients' waiting room and the other to an internal corridor that leads to the staff room, where the doctors who supervise the medical trainees are located. This enables doctors to move from the consulting rooms to the supervisors' room easily and unobserved by the patients in the waiting room. During my research it also enabled me to switch the

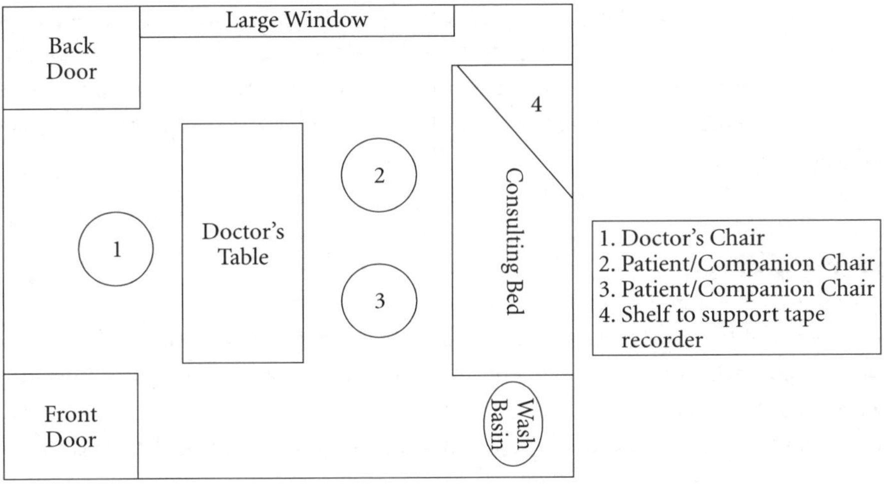

Figure 1. Consulting room 1

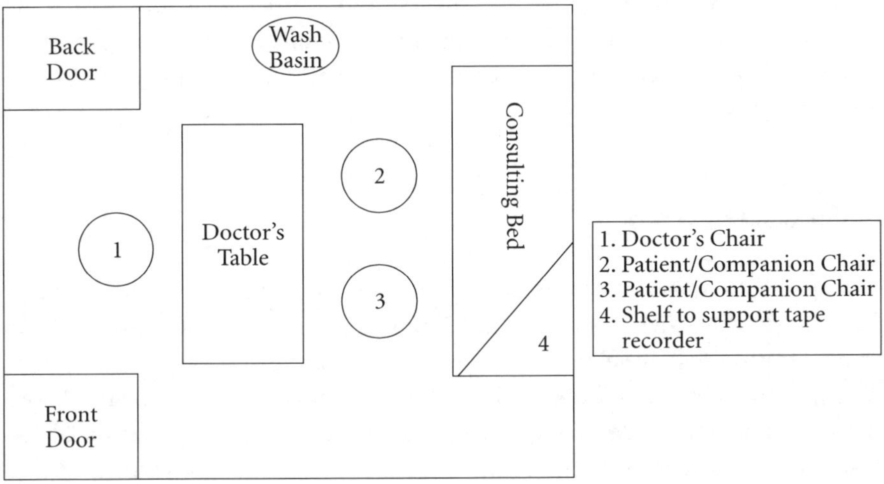

Figure 2. Consulting room 2

tape-recorder discreetly on and off when the consulting room was empty. Each consulting room was furnished with a wooden desk, two chairs, a bed, and a basin (see Figures 1 and 2).

A tape-recorder stand was built into the corner of each consulting room used for this study. The corner closest to the bed was chosen since this was facing the patient's back. Because of the design of the consulting rooms, it was decided to hang a personal clip microphone to the ceiling to obtain maximum clarity of sound. The microphone was placed above eye level to avoid any discomfort to either doctor or patient. A portable Marantz cassette recorder PMD 222 was used for this study as its pitch, tone and decibel controller made for a better quality recording than the standard tape-recorder with a personal microphone.

3.6 Permissions

The first step towards gaining permission to carry out my research in the Clinic was to make administrators at the Pontificia Universidad Católica de Chile and scholars at its Faculty of Medicine aware of the potential contribution that the study could make to the work of the institution and to the understanding of medical discourse generally.

Contacts in Chile were initiated two years before the recording of data took place in order to ascertain and meet the ethical requirements of the PUC, as principal institution, and of the San Joaquín Outpatient Clinic where the research was to be conducted (see Appendices 5 and 6). During this time, I also provided the documentation required by the Ethics Committee of Monash University, my home institution.

3.7 Stage I: Observation

During the first few weeks of fieldwork I held meetings with the Dean of the Faculty of Medicine, the Medical Head of the Outpatient Clinic and the administration personnel of PUC to learn more about the structure and functioning of the Clinic, and about the public health system in Santiago. Before any recording was undertaken, I spent some time observing how social exchanges were conducted in the Clinic, which helped me to choose the language style and behaviour that were appropriate and which would encourage people to co-operate in the project. It was critical that respect and friendliness were shown to everyone involved. On my arrival in Chile I had to overcome some initial obstacles before winning the support of the participants in this project. Refining the paralinguistic and linguistic aspects of communication proved to be the crucial key to being accepted by doctors, administrators, secretaries and patients of the institution.

Following the example of Corsaro (1982), I also involved the *auxiliares*, the assistant nurses, who worked in the Clinic and who were responsible for the allocation of doctors to the seven consulting rooms. With their co-operation, I was able to arrange for those doctors who were taking part in the project to be allocated to the two consulting rooms equipped with the recording facilities required for this study.

There are a number of procedures that a patient follows before seeing a doctor. The regulations provide either for the patient to choose a particular doctor or for one of the doctors on duty to be assigned to the patient. On the day of the consultation, the patient provides the assistant nurse with the receipt, *bono*, which indicates that the consultation has already been paid for. The assistant nurse then weighs the patient and records the information on the patient's medical card. Patients then wait to be called to the consulting room. The average waiting time is twenty minutes; however, this may be much longer if a doctor encounters difficulties in a consultation, patients do not arrive on time, or an emergency occurs.

3.8 Stage II: Questionnaire

The purpose of the questionnaire was to gather demographic information about the participants. This information was important when deciding which tapes would be transcribed and studied.

After agreeing to take part in the study, each participant completed one of two questionnaires before the consultation: the one designed for doctors (see Appendix 3) or the one for patients (see Appendix 2). Doctors were required to give their age, sex, years of medical practice and nationality.[3] Patients gave their age, sex, occupation and nationality. Information about each patient's number of visits to the Clinic and their familiarity with medical procedures in the Clinic was also requested.

3.9 Stage III: Semi-structured interview

The aim of the semi-structured interview was to gain an understanding of patients' attitudes towards doctors and to find out whether patients' opinions were then revealed in the consultation. Using an ethnographic approach to discourse analysis, patients were asked what it was they liked and disliked about their doctor. These two questions were added as a result of the patients' own interest in the topic, as I realized soon after talking to patients that they would spontaneously initiate a conversation about their likes and dislikes of the medical system and of the doctors in the Clinic.

A total of 134 patients contributed to the semi-structured interview process. Patients were allowed to give extensive answers which were transcribed verbatim so as to keep an accurate record of their views. Completing each semi-structured interview took between 20 and 30 minutes.

3.10 Stage IV: Tape-recording of the medical consultation

Tape-recording of the data was developed in two stages. A pilot study was carried out initially, which served to improve the final design for the recording of the data to be used in the analysis.

The pilot study was undertaken during the first few weeks of September 1997 in order to determine the best location for the tape-recorder and to select the best consulting rooms for recording purposes. At this stage any doctor or patient willing to participate could be involved, which meant that participants knew they were collaborating in a trial and that their recording was not part of the data designed to be transcribed or analysed in any way. These volunteers were asked to give any feedback (at the end of the consultation) that could help to achieve the most naturalistic recording in a way that would not interfere with the medical interview. After a number of trials it became clear that patients were uncomfortable with a tape-recorder visible on the doctor's desk. The solution therefore was to place the tape-recorder in a corner of the consulting room. All consultations were recorded in the morning sessions.

3.11 The participants

3.11.1 The researcher

Since this research has an ethnographic approach to discourse analysis, a description of the researcher involved is necessary. The researcher is a Chilean-born female with a middle-class background who was in her mid-thirties at the time of the recording. She completed primary, secondary and tertiary education in Chile, lived for three years in Italy, and then established herself in Australia in 1988 where she completed postgraduate studies. The researcher's role in the study was primarily one of observer; however, she also conducted the questionnaire and the semi-structured interview, and maintained regular contact with medical and general staff, including participating in their social and academic activities. The involvement of the researcher in the tape-recording was not noticed by either the doctor or the patient, since she used the back door to get in and out the consulting rooms when changing tapes. This meant that the researcher was never in the consulting room when the doctor and the patient entered the room.

3.11.2 The doctors

This section describes the profiles of doctors who were involved in Stages II and IV of the study.

Stage II
Three of the six doctors who completed the questionnaire were females who had completed their primary, secondary and tertiary education in Chile. They were in their late twenties/early thirties and had completed no more than two years of medical practice. The three male doctors had also been educated entirely in Chile. Two were in their late thirties/early forties and had ten or more years' medical experience. The third male doctor was in his late twenties and had been practising medicine for less than a year.

Stage IV
The analysis involved tape-recorded consultations of four of these six doctors: two females (Dr. Ana and Dr. Berta[4]) and two males (Dr. Carlos and Dr. Daniel) (see Table 2). The two male doctors were those with more than ten years' medical experience. The other two doctors were excluded from this

Table 2. Profile of doctors in tape-recorded consultations

Name	Sex	Age group	Number of years' medical experience
Dr. Ana	F	25–35	< 2 years
Dr. Berta	F	25–35	< 2 years
Dr. Carlos	M	36–45	> 10 years
Dr. Daniel	M	36–45	> 10 years

Table 3. Age distribution of female and male patients completing the questionnaire

Patient's age	< 20	21–30	31–40	41–50	51–60	61–70	71+
Females	7	9	14	23	15	21	7
Males	1	3	6	3	10	12	3

study because they attended patients who did not match the selection criteria for inclusion in the analysis.

Since the ages and experience of the male doctors did not match those of the female doctors, the emergence of linguistic differences must be interpreted with caution, as gender effects may be confounded by the effects of age/experience (see Cicourel 1995). This is the reason why the analysis has not placed greater emphasis on gender as a variable in the discourse. General patterns suggesting a male or female speaker are presented as appropriate, but these remain secondary to a more detailed investigation of the other demographic factors outlined above.

3.11.3 The patients

This section describes the patients who participated in Stages II, III and IV.

Stage II

The total number of patients who completed the questionnaire was 134: 96 females and 38 males. They ranged in age from 15 to 87 years, and included professionals, tradesmen, students, house managers and retirees. Women in their forties and sixties made up the largest group of female patients (61.4%), while men in their fifties and sixties comprised the majority of male patients (58.6%). Those aged either 20 or less or 71 and over formed the smallest groups for both sexes – and were also the two categories which consulted their doctor least often. Interestingly, female patients visited their doctor almost three times more often than males. The age and sex of the patients are set out in Table 3.

According to information obtained from the hospital administration in January 1998, participants in this study were mostly in the public health system (FONASA).

Stage III

The patients who were involved in the semi-structured interview were the same as those who had completed the questionnaire (Stage II).

Stage IV

Of the 134 individuals who had completed the questionnaire, more than 100 gave permission to tape-record their consultation. After a careful selection process (explained below), 22 were chosen for the study. In order that comparisons of patients' discourse were meaningful it was important to gather information from a group who shared socio-demographic similarities. I selected the age group that was most prominently represented in the Clinic (information provided by Gerencia General PUC 1997). Teenagers and mature adult patients were therefore excluded. Participants were also controlled on the basis of the number of visits they had made to the same doctor in the Clinic. Those familiar with the procedures were included, while those visiting the Centre for the first time were not.

My selection of the recorded material also took into consideration the number of people involved in the medical interview. Specifically, I discounted consultations involving third persons; for example, many mature-age patients and young persons were frequently accompanied by family members. These consultations also tended to involve patients who were visiting the Clinic for the first time. In addition, recordings were rejected when the sound quality was poor due to echo resonance or when the voices were not clearly differentiated because of external noise. Noise problems severely hampered transcription of the data and led to many untranscribed sequences.

The composition of each doctor–patient dyad is given in Tables 4 to 7. Again, patients are referred to by pseudonyms throughout to protect their privacy. Each table lists the patient's name, age group and occupation, and their consulting doctor. Overall, the youngest patients in the study were in the 31–40 age group (Alicia, Flavio and Paola) and the oldest was in her seventies (Yolanda). The other 18 patients were in their 40s, 50s or 60s.

Table 4. Profile of female patients consulting female doctors

Name	Age	Occupation	Doctor
Alicia	31–40	Home duties & student	Dr. Ana
Beatriz	51–60	Home duties	Dr. Ana
Carmen	41–50	Secretary	Dr. Ana
Gina	51–60	Secretary	Dr. Berta
Hilda	61–70	Accountant	Dr. Berta
Javiera	61–70	Home duties	Dr. Berta

Table 5. Profile of male patients consulting female doctors*

Name	Age	Occupation	Doctor
David	41–50	Publisher	Dr. Ana
Esteban	51–60	Worker	Dr. Ana
Flavio	31–40	Engineer	Dr. Ana

* Dr. Berta did not attend any of the male patients in the study. This situation arose principally because most of her male patients were first-time visitors and so were not familiar with the PUC Clinic.

Table 6. Profile of male patients consulting male doctors

Name	Age	Occupation	Doctor
Leonel	61–70	Butler	Dr. Carlos
Manuel	61–70	Worker	Dr. Carlos
Nicolás	61–70	Pensioner	Dr. Daniel
Samuel	61–70	(not provided)	Dr. Daniel
Tito	41–50	Assistant	Dr. Daniel
Victor	41–50	Mechanic	Dr. Daniel

Table 7. Profile of female patients consulting male doctors

Name	Age	Occupation	Doctor
Olga	41–50	Home duties	Dr. Carlos
Paola	31–40	Secretary	Dr. Carlos
Rosa	41–50	Home duties	Dr. Carlos
Wilma	41–50	Home duties	Dr. Daniel
Ximena	41–50	Accountant	Dr. Daniel
Yolanda	71–80	Home duties	Dr. Daniel
Zenobia	61–70	Home duties	Dr. Daniel

3.12 Data analysis

Preliminary data from the questionnaires (Stage II) was drawn on to select the 22 patients participating in the study. The semi-structured interview (Stage III) provided information on what patients liked and did not like about doctors and complemented the data obtained from the tape-recorded consultations (Stage IV). Subsequently, this information was categorized according to key themes that were found to emerge.

The analysis of the tape-recorded data involved 22 consultations. The data was transcribed using a selective number of transcript symbols following Du Bois. He writes:

> Discourse transcription can be defined as the process of creating a representation in writing of a speech event so as to make it accessible to discourse research. (1991:72)

This means that the system of transcription needs to be based on "what kind of research questions one seeks to answer" (Du Bois 1991:72). Similarly, Ochs (1979) argues that the transcription design is bound to the theoretical framework of the analysis rather than simply a mechanical written reproduction of the speech. Thus, "the transcript should reflect the particular interests – the hypotheses to be examined – of the researcher" (Ochs 1979:44). The transcription system in this study therefore includes those Du Bois symbols which were relevant to the data analysis and which would aid in answering the research questions being asked.

Some of the transcript symbols were modified to accommodate the Spanish data (see Appendix 4). For example, Du Bois's truncated intonation unit has been expanded in order to differentiate between Spanish conventional last truncated syllable with the symbol ' (e.g. *pa'* for *para*, "for" or "to") and the middle and final truncated syllable with the symbol – (e.g. *Uste–* for *Usted*, "you"). The symbols ¿¡ were added to the classification of transitional continuity to be consistent with the Spanish first and end position of appeal and exclamation markers (e.g. *¿cómo está?*, "how are you?"; *¡hola!*, "hi!"). Capital letters were also added to indicate that the voice quality of the speaker was loud and emphatic (e.g. *AHORA*, "NOW". The symbol to show vowel elongation differs from that used by Du Bois. In this study the lengthening of a vowel is normally shown by a colon (e.g. *pero:*, "but"), but in some cases the lengthening is longer and it is represented by double colons (e.g. *pero::*). The symbol = (used by Du Bois to represent vowel lengthening) indicates here that no pause has been left between the last word uttered by the first speaker and the first word uttered by the second speaker. This is referred to by Sacks et al. (1974) as *latching* and concords with Coates, for whom "an equals sign at the end of one speaker's utterance and at the start of the next utterance indicates the absence of a discernable gap" (1996: xiii). In order to retain the authenticity of the speech, the transcription preserves the natural and unpolished spoken language.

Pauwels (1995) has identified a number of communication routines commonly used by health professionals during the medical consultation. These include *Greeting and introduction*, *History-taking*, *Explanations and instruction during physical examinations*, *Management and treatment of a health problem or health issue* and *Prevention*. Greetings and introductions were excluded from this study because the initiation of communication usually started in the waiting room where the patient's name would be called out by the doctor. The two would then exchange greetings while they were walking into the consulting room where the recording was to take place. Physical examination as part of the history-taking routine was also excluded because it took place too far away from the microphone and the quality of the recordings was poor. This also meant that the prescription stage could not be included since it could not be linked to the talk that preceded it. Therefore, the data selected for analysis in this study is taken from:

a. The discourse developed in follow-up visits to the Clinic by the 22 patients during the history-taking routine.
b. The management and treatment of these patients' health problems, including assessment of test results.

The following examples from the present study demonstrate these communication routines of medical discourse in practice. History-taking may involve:-

The doctor's summary of the last visit:

Example 1 Consultation Nº 15 (Doctor: Carlos, Patient: Rosa)

13 D: … *la última vez que nos vimos fue el veintidós de agosto*
the last time we saw each other was 22 August

…

15 D: … *nos vimos porque estaba bajo un tratamiento por un*
we saw each other because you were being treated

16 *cuadro depresivo*
for depression

Questioning by the doctor:

Example 2 Consultation Nº 5 (Doctor: Ana, Patient: Esteban)

10 D: *¿Cuénteme le han vuelto a dar esas crisis? ¿Se acuerda que*
Tell me, have you had these crises again lately? Do you remember that

11 *tenía como crisis de angustia? ¿Ahora son pequeños momentos de angustia?*
you used to have, as it were, crises of anxiety? Are they short periods of anxiety now?

Summaries and enquiries were usually followed by the doctor's assessment of the test results. Markers initiating the assessment include a statement of the medication or therapy previously prescribed, followed by an adjective or adverb.

Example 3 Consultation Nº 10 (Doctor: Carlos, Patient: Leonel)

56 D: *El antígeno prostático ... está funcionando O.K. ...*
The prostatic antigen ... is working O.K. ...

In these follow-up visits the conclusion of the management and treatment routine was marked by the doctor's request to carry out a physical examination, usually involving a check of the patient's blood pressure.

Example 4 Consultation Nº 9 (Doctor: Berta, Patient: Javiera)

48 D: ... *Vamos a ver como están las presione– ahora*
... We'll check to see how it is now

Example 5 Consultation Nº 12 (Doctor: Carlos, Patient: Nicolás)

500 D: ... *Descúbrase la camisa que le voy a ver dónde le duele*
... Open up your shirt so that I can see where you have the pain

3.13 The volume of data

Doctors used approximately 12,829 words in total in the 22 consultations recorded, a number almost identical to that used by patients, namely 12,923 words (see Appendix 1). The mean number of words for doctors (both male and female) per conversation was 583.1 (±505.4 Standard Deviation, n = 22 conversations) and the mean number of words per patient per conversation was 587.4 (±361.8, n = 22). The difference is not significant (two-way

ANOVA: $F_{1,36} = 0.128$, $P = 0.722$). Moreover, there is no significant difference in the word count for history-taking or management and treatment between the four doctor–patient dyads ($F_{3,36} = 0.553$, $P = 0.649$), nor any significant differences between each doctor–patient dyad and the communication routine ($F_{3,36} = 0.537$, $P = 0.659$). This analysis reveals that both doctors and patients used a remarkably similar number of words in the discourse and suggests that both participants had the opportunity to take the floor during the consultation and to elaborate on their speech. In order to fully understand this process, a deconstruction of doctors' and patients' talk into distinctive *voices* has been undertaken.

3.14 *Voices* in doctor–patient communication

During the history-taking and management and treatment routines, doctors use different forms of talk as they conduct the consultation. Patients also adopt different forms of talk in the course of the medical visit. In this study, these forms of talk are referred to as *voices.*

3.14.1 Analysis of doctors' *voices*

The analysis identified three distinct *voices* used by doctors in medical discourse, which I have called here the *Doctor voice*, *Educator voice* and *Fellow Human voice.* These distinctions enable us to focus more precisely on what it is that physicians *do* in their medical talk and to understand the relationship that exists between a particular *voice* and its interactional accomplishment. The three *voices* correspond to the three functional medical goals identified by Cohen-Cole (1991:4) as

a. Gathering information about the patient's health.
b. Educating the patient to adhere to a medical recommendation.
c. Providing support and showing empathy.

The *Doctor voice* recalls details of the previous visit and finds out how the patient has been faring by asking a number of questions. These usually relate to the patient's symptoms, tests or treatment ordered, medication, compliance, lifestyle and so on, and can take various discourse forms. This function of the *Doctor voice* we will term *Seeking information.* A second function, *Assessment and review,* occurs in the management and treatment routine of the follow-up visit. Here the doctor studies the test results ordered at the previous consultation, assesses the need for further tests or treatment, and determines whether the patient has been compliant with earlier instructions. A third function of the *Doctor voice* is to assert the expected roles and obligations of each participant in the exchange; in particular, the doctor's role of questioning the patient about his/her health and dictating various actions that should be undertaken, and the patient's role of providing information that will assist in ongoing management and showing compliance with the doctor's requests. In this process, the socio-cultural background of each participant is often revealed, and doctors may show an alignment to the medical institution and their profession. Accordingly, this function has been designated *Alignment to authority*.

The *Educator voice* reports various kinds of medical information to patients in the hope that a better understanding of their health problem and management will assist compliance. The information may outline the cause of the symptoms, the reasons for taking a certain medication or undergoing a procedure; this *voice* also responds to accounts of patient discomfort. In my analysis I am particularly interested in those linguistic functions and forms and discourse strategies that serve to provide patients with the knowledge that will enable them to better comprehend the requirements and responsibilities of managing their illness.

The *Doctor* and *Educator voices* define medical discourse as different from other forms of talk, as one participant is the expert who seeks information, provides treatment, educates and commands authority, while the other participant provides information, complies with treatment, becomes educated and respects authority. These *voices* therefore operate within the asymmetrical framework of the institution discussed in Chapter 2.

The *Fellow Human voice* differs from the other two *voices* in that its utterances more closely resemble everyday talk, which, as we noted in the previous chapter, does not seek an elevated role or require any special expertise in order to be carried out successfully, though it is required to display socio-cultural competence (Hymes 1972) by knowing how to interact with the patient in a way that develops empathy. This *voice* differs from the *Doctor voice* and the *Educator voice* in that it is likely to be linked to an affiliative discourse (Davis 1988) that is both friendly and co-operative (Schiffrin 1984). It is difficult to document all the linguistic features and strategies associated with the *Fellow Human voice*. However, this study explores a number of functions involved in the performance of this *voice* and a range of discourse forms used to achieve an empathic and affiliative communication.

3.14.2 Analysis of patients' *voices*

The analysis of patients' discourse aims to identify what it is that patients *do* during the medical consultation, how they present themselves, and whether they see the consultation as an opportunity to develop their stories. Clearly, in contrast to doctors, patients have not been formally trained for their "role" as patients and do not bring to the consultation a structural framework for their forms of talk. Nonetheless, it is possible to distinguish the *voice* of *Health-related storytelling*, the *voice* of *Competence* and the *voice* of *Social communicator* in their speech as they discuss their health condition, their experiences with medical treatment, their families or job situations, or indeed any event they consider relevant to their presentation at the Clinic. In addition, the *voice* of *Initiator* challenges the findings of some studies that patients are passive entities who merely respond to physicians' questions (West 1984; Bergman 1992), lack initiative (West 1984), and accept, without hesitation, any decision offered to them by their care providers (Blanchard et al. 1988).

It is the aim of my analysis to hear what patients have to *say* during the consultation as well as what they *do* in response to physicians' talk. That is, I am interested in the contributions patients make to the discourse and the ways in which their *voices* interact with doctors' *voices*. I am also interested in whether patients' *voices* reflect, reinforce or contest the inherent asymmetry of the institutional exchange.

3.14.3 Limitations to the number of *voices*

It could be argued that the number of *voices* included in my analysis does not represent all possible *voices* in medical discourse. In recognizing this limitation, attention is drawn to Sinclair and Coulthard's criteria for descriptive analysis (1975: 15–17); these were adopted by Stubbs (1983) in his study of the meta-communicative functions performed by a teacher when interacting with students in a classroom situation, and have been drawn on in the present analysis. Sinclair and Coulthard's criteria are:

a. Incorporation of further descriptive categories should be allowed.
b. Descriptive categories need to be connected to the data in order to avoid repeating classifications.
c. Descriptive analysis should be used throughout the transcript.
d. Descriptions should share structural similarities and constraints.

In this research, the number of *voices* could have been expanded by making even finer distinctions in each of the main *voices*. However, each of the four patient *voices* can be identified in terms of the subject being developed in the conversation, with the *voice* of *Competence* further divided into three descriptive categories. Likewise, the three *voices* assigned to the doctors' performance are comprehensive of the forms of talk used in the consultation and also correspond to Cohen-Cole's three functional goals of the medical visit set out above.

Utterances were carefully classified in terms of their linguistic form and categorized according to the structural similarities of grammar or communicative function (Gumperz 1982b). This process was complex and delicate owing to the multi-functionality of utterances. While some could be easily classified (e.g. questions asking for information), others required a functional and contextual interpretation for correct identification (e.g. questions embedded in a patient's narrative). In order to prevent the problem of classifying the same utterance twice, those utterances that had the same communicative function were first codified and then investigated to see whether there was a linguistic form that could be identified in them.

The frequency of each *voice* in the medical discourse and the frequency of each function within that *voice* will be documented. Analyses will outline the most prominent features emerging from the data.

3.15 Ethical issues

This study shares Cameron's view that "empowering research must give attention to the research process as well as the research product" (1992: 121). All participants were freely involved in the research process. As set out in the Explanatory Statement (Appendix 5), they had the right to listen to their recording, and could withdraw their consent at any time if they wished to do so without this affecting them in any way. The information gathered was strictly confidential and the real names of doctors and patients have been changed. In addition, personal information such as patients' addresses and citizen identification numbers given during the consultation has been suppressed. Participants signed a consent form (Appendix 6) after reading the Explanatory Statement or after they were asked to give permission to tape-record their linguistic contribution to the medical interview.

Since the completion of this research I have conducted a series of seminars addressed to both medical doctors and linguistic colleagues to share with them the findings of this study. Again, I agree strongly with Cameron (1992) that the knowledge acquired in any research into discourse patterns should be fed back into the community that provided the information for the study, so that there is a "redistribution [of] knowledge" (Cameron 1992: 119). According to Cameron, "speakers themselves should possess the relevant information and the analytic tools to make use of it in ways which they determine" (1992: 118).

The study was approved by the Standing Committee on Ethics in Research on Humans, Monash University (date: 1996, project number: 258/95); by the Doctors' Committee of the *Pontificia Universidad Católica de Chile* (letter dated 20 September 1995); and by the Head of General Practice in the *Centro de Diagnóstico de la Universidad Católica de Chile* (verbal communication, September 1997).

Notes

1. Personal communication from Mr. Enrique Mena, Manager of the PUC Outpatient Clinic, December 1997.

2. Information kindly provided by the General Adminstration of the San Joaquín Outpatient Clinic.

3. Nationality can be a controversial aspect of a person's identity. In this study, all doctors and patients claimed Chilean nationality, coinciding with the country where they had lived all their lives.

4. Chilean socio-cultural pragmatics requires doctors to be addressed by their surname. However, first names are used in this study to indicate gender. Pseudonyms have also been used in order to maintain confidentiality and anonymity.

Chapter 4

The *Doctor voice*

This chapter explores the first of the three doctor *voices* that were introduced in Section 3.14 as they function in the communication routines of (1) history-taking and (2) management and treatment of a health problem or health issue (Pauwels 1995), and specifically in the context of follow-up visits. In the previous chapter, the three functions identified with the *Doctor voice* were introduced: *Seeking information*, *Assessment and review*, and *Alignment to authority*. These functions will now be investigated in turn, describing the different discourse strategies associated with each function and illustrating their usage through extracts from the transcripts. The frequency of each function and strategy is summarized in statistical tables in order to highlight individual preferences among the four doctors of the study and to note whether there were any significant variations in the findings along gender lines.

4.1 Seeking information

Physicians assume the *Doctor voice* in order to find out informative data about the patient's health condition that will enable them to make a diagnosis and/or to assess changes that may have occurred since the previous visit. In this section I analyse the discourse strategies associated with this function. Questions seeking information (QSI) are categorized as *QSI one* (only one question asked), *QSI chain* (a string of questions), *QSI multiple choice*, *QSI Recycling/Repetition*, and *QSI+Summary/Summary+QSI*. The forms and functions of each category are analysed as they occur in specific examples.

Several instances were recorded during the history-taking and management routines in which doctors asked only one question to ascertain the patient's health condition (*QSI one*). In the following extract the female patient tells her doctor that she has been experiencing stomach aches and diarrhoea every evening before returning home from work.

Example 6 Consultation Nº 3 (Doctor: Ana, Patient: Carmen)

23 D: *Ya y eso ¿desde cuándo que está con esa mo[lestia?]*
Right, and since when have you been feeling that dis[comfort?]

24 P: *[Desde] digamo– desde que*
[Since] let's say since I

25 *empecé ma– o meno– con ésto*
more or less started with this

26 D: *Ya*
O.K.

The *QSI one* used by Dr. Ana – *¿desde cuándo que está con esa molestia?* – seeks information about the time period that Carmen has been feeling unwell (i.e. symptoms of nausea and diarrhoea). This is introduced by *desde* ("since"), a temporal conjunction. However, Carmen does not provide an answer that relates to time, such as "last week" or "two weeks ago". Instead she replies, *desde que empecé … con ésto. Esto* ("this") relates to her previous utterance in which she mentioned that her discomfort starts every evening when she is preparing to leave work for home. The doctor's minimal response is given by *Ya* ("O.K.")

From the analysis it is evident that *QSI one* questions could be further divided into those that are oriented towards the illness or ailment as such, and therefore relate primarily to specific medical information, and those that are intended to find out about the effect that the health condition may have or has had on the patient's life. In the next example, Olga indicates that she experiences difficulty in moving her right hand because of a bone and ligament problem. Dr. Carlos wants to know whether this has impeded her usual activities.

Example 7 Consultation Nº 13 (Doctor: Carlos, Patient: Olga)

329 D: *¿Hay alguna cosa que le agrade hacer sobre manera?*
Is there anything you really enjoy doing?

330 P: *Me fascina jardinear …*
I love gardening

331 D: *¿Y en este tiempo lo ha estado haciendo?*
Have you been doing it lately?

332 P: *… aunque esté cansa–a, cansa–a, cansa–a yo jardineo igual.*
… even if I'm feeling tired, tired, tired, I do the gardening nevertheless.

The patient has been having severe pain in her arm. Dr. Carlos uses a *QSI one* in line 331, *¿Y en este tiempo lo ha estado haciendo?*, to seek information about Olga's ability to carry out her favourite activity. This type of question reflects a more holistic approach to health, since the doctor could have uttered a *QSI* focusing on the pain of the body part (for example, *¿Tiene dolor en el brazo?*, "Do you have any pain in your arm?"), instead of asking about the effect the pain was having on his patient's life. This idea will be explored further in the chapter on the *Fellow Human voice.*

The *QSI chain* was also documented in this study. According to West (1984: 82), this type of questioning may reduce the chances of all of the questions being answered; indeed, the patient may respond to only one of the questions in the chain series. In the following extract the doctor asks three questions in succession.

Example 8 Consultation Nº 5 (Doctor: Ana, Patient: Esteban)

10 D: *¿Cuénteme le han vuelto a dar esas crisis? ¿Se acuerda que tenía como crisis*
Tell me, have you had these crises again lately? Do you remember that you used to have, as it were, crises

11 *de angustia? ¿Ahora son pequeños momentos de angustia?*
of anxiety? Are they short periods of anxiety now?

12 P: *Pequeños momentos de angustia sí.*
Short period of anxiety, yes.

Here all three questions refer to the patient's episodes of anxiety. The first question asks about any re-occurrence of the attacks, the second asks whether the patient can recall the earlier episodes, and the third asks for information on the current pattern of the illness. The temporal adverb *ahora* ("now") initiates the last question, which is made in the present tense. The patient's response is simply to echo the doctor's last utterance, confirming West's findings above. Thus, the *QSI chain* may be counterproductive as a strategy for eliciting information.

The category of *QSI multiple choice* comprises two discourse parts, in which the second part asks the opposite of the first, with the link between the two parts accomplished with the conjunction *o* ("or"). In Example 9 the doctor asks his patient to tell him whether the pain is present from the time he wakes up in the morning, or whether it is related to something in particular that he does during the day.

Example 9 Consultation Nº 12 (Doctor: Carlos, Patient: Nicolás)

211 D: *¿Cuándo está ese uh ese malestar?, ¿ocurre toda– la– mañana– al despertar?*
When you have this discomfort, does it happen every morning when you wake up?

212 *Uste– me decía ¿cuándo se pone nervioso o cuándo tiene que hacer algo?*
Or, as I think you said, is it when you feel tense or when you have to do something?

213 P: *Cuando me levanto yo de la cama yo me levanto completamente perfecto.*
When I get up I feel perfectly well.

214 *cuando YA salgo fuera de la casa ahí:=*
It's when I leave home that I get it:=

Dr. Carlos's multiple choice question proposes three alternatives that have been offered in a chain. Each alternative is introduced by the interrogative *cuándo* ("when"). The conjunction *o* ("or") and the elliptical verb form *ocurre* ("does it happen") are repeated in the second and third utterance. Thus, the doctor is asking the patient, "Does it [the discomfort] happen ... when you wake up ... when you feel tense ... or when you have to do something?" The patient's answer relates to the last option offered to him by the doctor and is produced with an intonation emphasis (*YA*) to indicate with force when it is that he feels under stress.

The use of recycled questions was also found in the data. Doctors may use *recycling/repetition* when the patient has not provided the information required. In this next extract we can see how the same question is reformulated later in the interview.

Example 10 Consultation Nº 13 (Doctor: Carlos, Patient: Olga)

479 D: *¿Uste– se nota que está más irritable de lo habitual, que explote con más*
Have you noticed that you are more irritable than usual, that you get angry more

480 *facilidad?*
easily?

...

485 D: *¿Las cosas que antes le irritaban ahora también le irritan?*
Do the things that irritated you in the past still make you irritable?

The comparative utterance *está más irritable de lo habitual* ("you are more irritable than usual") implies that the patient's behaviour may have changed from less irritable to more irritable. The reformulation in line 485 now includes two adverbs of time, *antes* ("before") and *ahora* ("now"), which work to contrast the pattern of the patient's irritability in the past and in the present. These questions help the doctor to ascertain whether the patient has given full and accurate information about her health status.

The data also included examples of a combination of *QSI* and summary components, i.e. *QSI+Summary* and *Summary+QSI*. In *QSI+Summary*, a *QSI* that seeks information about the patient's present state of health is followed by a summary that focuses on some relevant points already discussed, either in previous visits or earlier in the current consultation. In *Summary+QSI* the order is reversed. In both categories the *Summary* draws on the patient's history to provide a contextual framework for the doctor's question(s). The discourse forms of the *QSI+Summary* and *Summary+QSI* were found to be similar, with the patient's medical history always delivered in the past tense (preterite or imperfect). The following example illustrates a *QSI+Summary*.

Example 11 Consultation Nº 5 (Doctor: Ana, Patient: Esteban)

35 D: ...*¿Cuénteme como ha estado de ésto?*
Tell me how you have been with this?

36 *¿Se acuerda de la molestia que tenía en [la parte genital]?*
Do you remember you had discomfort in [your genital region]

37 P: *[Sí, sí, sí] Bien, bien=*
[Yes, yes, yes] Well, well=

38 D: *=Eso pasó totalmente*
=That's fully over

39 P: *con la gracia de Dios y a y a debido al trata tratam tratamiento suyo po'*
Thanks to God and your treat, treat, (medical) treatment

40 D: *Ya, o sea que bue/no\. Sí, lo tratamos como una micosis=*
That's good /no\. Yes, we treated (the case) as a mycosis=

41 P: *=<WH Sí WH>=*
=<WH Yes WH>=

42 D: *=y lo dejamos con eh Fungium por diez día–*
=and we prescribed Fungium for you (to be taken) for ten days

43 P: *Así es*
Yes, that's right

44 D: *Y si no seguíamos con el problema íbamos hacer un examen, un dermatológico*
And if it didn't work we had in mind to have a dermatological test

Here the doctor initiates her turn with a *QSI one* in line 35 asking the patient to report on his genital discomfort. Without waiting for his reply, she asks a second question in line 36 as an introduction to her summary of the patient's previous management and proposed alternative for ongoing treatment. Her summarizing helps to prompt the patient's memory and he contributes utterances of agreement after each of her statements.

Finally, we see two examples of a *Summary+QSI*.

Example 12 Consultation Nº 15 (Doctor: Carlos, Patient: Rosa)

29 D: *Vamo– a repasar un poco. Hoy día estamo– hace má– o meno– ocho meses*
We are going to review (your case) a little. Today we are. It's about eight months ago

30 *tuvo un conflicto con un sobrino*
that you had a row with your nephew

...

35 D: *Ya y eso la ha, la ha angustia–o ah: le ha quita–o el ánimo*
And (that's) upset you. It's taken away your energy

36 *[le ha quita–o gana de hacer cosa]*
[your wish to do things]

...

44 D: *¿Cuénteme qué medicamento está tomando?*
Tell me, what medication are you taking?

The doctor summarizes Rosa's last visit in lines 29–36 and then in line 44 asks if she is currently taking any medication. It is understood from the context that the medication in question is being used to treat her for emotional problems following the family argument.

Similarly, the doctor summarizes the information the patient had already provided during the consultation to introduce a question:

Example 13 Consultation Nº 13 (Doctor: Carlos, Patient: Olga)

317 D: *El ánimo Uste– me dice que está malo ¿desde hace cuánto tiempo ... que está*
You're telling me that you feel low in spirits. How long ... have you felt

318 *malo?*
low?

Table 8 summarizes the relative frequencies of the five *QSI* categories. *QSI one* is clearly the discourse strategy most widely used to gather information, ac-

Table 8. Discourse strategies used in *Seeking information*: summary

Discourse strategy	Frequency	%
QSI one	249	70.0
QSI chain	25	7.0
QSI multiple choice	42	11.8
QSI Recycling/Repetition	19	5.3
QSI+Summary/Summary+QSI	21	5.9
TOTAL	356	100

counting for 70% of the total. A distant second is *QSI multiple choice* with 11.8%. Other discourse strategies were used even less frequently.

Table 9 provides a more detailed account of the data, giving individual results for each of the four doctors and dividing the patients into male and female. The most obvious pattern to emerge from these doctor–patient dyads is the high frequency of *QSI one* usage by Dr. Carlos, with the gender of the patient having no apparent effect (68 and 61), contrasting with his relatively high use of *QSI multiple choice* when interviewing male patients (17). It is possible that this reflects an idiosyncratic trait, or could perhaps be explained by Dr. Carlos's age and/or the particular medical condition of his patients; however, there is no strong evidence to support these suppositions. We can observe, too, that Dr. Carlos asked the most number of questions in each category, as well as the most overall (187). Notable also is that, while *QSI one* was the preferred type of questioning of all four doctors, Dr. Daniel differed from the others in asking his female patients a disproportionate number of *QSI ones* (34) compared to males (16). Three of these women were housewives and all were over 40, but their ages varied widely. Whether socio-demographic factors contributed to this gender bias is a question that needs further investigation. The other categories were spread fairly evenly.

4.2 Assessment and review

The physician also assumes the *Doctor voice* when making an assessment of test results or treatment that was recommended at the previous visit, and as part of reviewing the patient's compliance and progress with that treatment. This section explores these two linguistic stages of the medical consultation.

Doctors sometimes initiate the discourse of the assessment with a summary of the previous visit. Unlike the *QSI* summaries described above, however, which are designed to refresh the patient's memory in order to frame the

Table 9. Discourse strategies used in *Seeking information*: frequencies for individual doctors and male/female patients

Discourse strategy	Dr. Ana Dr. Ana		Dr. Berta	Dr. Carlos		Dr. Daniel Dr. Daniel		TOTAL
	F (n=3)	M (n=3)	F (n=3)	F (n=3)	M (n=3)	F (n=4)	M (n=3)	
QSI one								
N	29	26	15	68	61	34	16	249
M	9.6	8.6	5.0	22.6	20.3	8.5	5.3	70.0%
QSI chain								
N	5	2	3	5	4	4	2	25
M	1.6	0.6	1.0	1.6	1.3	1.0	0.6	7.0%
QSI multiple choice								
N	6	3	1	6	17	3	6	42
M	2.0	1.0	0.3	2.0	5.6	0.7	2.0	11.8%
QSI Recycling/Repetition								
N	1	2	0	6	7	2	1	19
M	0.3	0.6	0.0	2.0	2.3	0.5	0.3	5.3%
QSI+Summary/Summary+QSI								
N	4	2	0	8	5	1	1	21
M	1.3	0.6	0.0	2.6	1.6	0.2	0.3	5.9%
TOTAL	45	35	19	93	94	44	26	356 100%

n = number of consultations; N = frequency; M = mean frequency per consultation question(s), the purpose of these assessment summaries is to provide a context for new information, such as telling the patient the test results or proposing to modify the treatment. These summaries often serve as the starting-point for the follow-up interview as a whole.

Example 14 Consultation Nº 15 (Doctor: Carlos, Patient: Rosa)

13 D: *A ver la última vez que nos vimos fue el veintidós de agosto*
Let's see, the last time we saw each other was 22 August

14 P: *Sí=*
Yes=

15 D: *=Ya, ahí estamos, nos vimos porque estaba bajo un tratamiento por un*
=O.K. here we are, we saw each other because you were being

16 *cuadro depresivo=*
treated for depression=

17 P: *=Sí=*
=Yes=

18 D: *=Y un trastorno digestivo=*
=And a digestive problem=

19 P: *=Sí=*
=Yes=

20 D: *=Este reflujo de presofágico=*
=This oesophageal reflux=

21 P: *=Sí*
=Yes

We can see in this extract that the doctor is describing the patient's medical history. The summary begins by indicating the date of the last consultation and continues by enumerating the medical problems the patient had at the time.

Patients at the Clinic usually brought their test results to the follow-up visit. These were then interpreted by the doctor and discussed with the patient. The discourse form of the assessment was found to be similar for each of the doctors. It was built around the verb *estar* ("to be"), indicating that the current test results indicated a particular health state. This was accompanied by an adjective that described *bien* ("good") or *mal* ("bad") results. In the data the doctors were able to describe any test result by making one comment only. This meant that all the tests they examined had common descriptive attributes. The example below illustrates this phenomenon.

Example 15 Consultation N° 12 (Doctor: Carlos, Patient: Nicolás)

424 D: ... *Están bastante mejor los exámenes*
... Your test results are considerably better

Here the doctor summarizes his assessment in a comparative form. The adjective *mejor* ("better"), preceded by the adverb of manner *bastante* ("considerably"), signals an emphatic comparison, underlining the fact that the previous results were not as "good" as the ones being discussed currently.

Doctors may also choose to enumerate every test conducted on the patient and make individual assessments. This is demonstrated in the next example.

Example 16 Consultation N° 10 (Doctor: Carlos, Patient: Leonel)

54 D: *El antígeno prostático ... está funcionando O.K. Está bien, no hay*
The prostatic antigen is working O.K. It's O.K. There's no

55 *problema. Listo. El examen de sangre ... [está]*
problem. All right. The blood test ... [is]

56 P: *[¿Ah sí?]*
[Oh! Yes?]

57 D: *En buena– condiciones=*
It's good=

58 P: *=O sea está normal=*
=Or rather, it's normal=

59 D: *=Está normal. El eloctrocardiograma, impecable=*
=It's normal. The electrocardiogram impeccable=

60 P: *=Ya=*
=O.K.=

61 D: *=Todavía no pasan balas por ahí=*
=It is still bullet-proof=

Dr. Carlos makes his assessment by beginning each utterance with the name of the test (the subject) followed by the verb *estar* ("to be"), used either explicitly (*El antígeno prostático está funcionando O.K.*) or elliptically (*El electrocardiograma, impecable*). The assessment includes not only an adjectival phrase (*en buenas condiciones*, "it's good") and adverbs like *bien* and *impecable* to describe the results, but also a metaphor: the ECG presents no trace of anomalies and is described as "still bullet-proof"; that is, impervious to damage.[1] However, the use of the adverb *todavía* ("still") also suggests the temporality of the patient's well-being and may indirectly bring to the surface his age (between 60 and 70), a reminder that such good health ought not be taken for granted (see Cordella 1999).

The *Doctor voice* also reviews whether the patient has understood how to follow the treatment prescribed at the previous visit and been compliant with the doctor's instructions. Sometimes the feedback or commentary on the patient's answers is minimal, as in the following extract.

Example 17 Consultation Nº 12 (Doctor: Carlos, Patient: Nicolás)

74 D: *¿Ha estado tomando el Lispor?*
Have you been taking the Lispor?

75 P: *... Eh: eh: es que me tomo el coktail en la mañana*
... Eh: eh: I take a cocktail (of medicines) in the morning

76 D: *Ya*
O.K.

77 P: *Lo– tre– que tomo Fluoxetina, y lo– do– el Lispor y no sé:*
I take three Fluoxetina, and the two Lispor, and, as for the rest, I don't know:

78 D: *Nitrendipino*
Nitrendipino

79 P: *El que me dió Uste–*
The one you gave me

80 D: *Ya y¿el Alopurinol lo sigue tomando?*
Yes. And are you still taking the Alopurinol?

81 P: *No*
No

82 D: *Ya, y la ¿Ranitidina?*
O.K., and the Ranitidina?

83 P: *Esa la tomo en la noche ...*
I take that one at night ...

84 D: *¡Ah la Ranitidina!=*
Ah the Ranitidina!=

85 P: *=Uhm=*
=Uhm=

86 D: *=Ya=*
=O.K.=

This sequence begins with a *QSI one* in line 74, the function of which is to assess the patient's compliance with taking the particular medicine Lispor. The progressive form of the verb (*Ha estado tomando*, "Have you been taking") emphasizes that the action should have started in the past and be continuing in the present. With this question the doctor hopes to ascertain the period of time the Lispor has been taken. In line 78 the question is in elliptical form, with only the name of the medicine mentioned. On the four occasions the doctor asks if the patient has been taking a prescribed medication (lines 74, 78, 80 and 82), he uses the minimal feedback sign *Ya* ("O.K./Yes") after the patient's reply. It features on its own in lines 76 and 86 and accompanies a question in lines 80 and 82.

As an example of a history-taking routine, we can see that the doctor's focus is on checking quickly through the list of previously prescribed medicines. At this stage he does not ask the patient to account for his non-compliance with Alopurinol or to describe the effects of his other medications. Later in the discourse, however, in the management and treatment routine, Dr. Carlos recalls the Alopurinol and asks Nicolás to stop taking it, because *no lo estaba tomando* ("you are not taking it")! We might wonder here that the doctor feels the need to *legitimize* what is already a matter of fact from the patient's perspective, while, at the same time, feeling no apparent need to enquire about the reason for the patient's decision to stop taking the Alopurinol.

The following example illustrates a different response when the test result for the patient indicates compliance with the medical recommendation. Here the discourse goes beyond the minimal feedback evident in the previous exchange.

Example 18 Consultation N° 18 (Doctor: Daniel, Patient: Victor)

74 D: … *Con la glicemia que trae (exámenes) lleva en forma muy correcta el*
… The result of the glycemia test shows that you're following your

75 *régimen* …
diet perfectly …

The use of the present tense of *lleva* ("to follow") stresses the certainty that the patient is following his diet properly, and this is then further accentuated by the intensifier *muy* ("very") that precedes the descriptive adjective *correcta* ("correct"). The utterance could also be interpreted as a compliment (see Cordella et al. 1995 for the use of compliments in Spanish) to a patient who is clearly competent in the management of his health problem.

The data showed that those patients who complied with a medical recommendation did not always receive this positive feedback. Instead, in some cases the doctor put a series of *QSI* to the patient without returning even a minimal response. This accords with the post-answer assessment studied by Jones (2001), who found that physicians rarely offered a commentary after patients provided newsworthy information during data collection. This contrasted with patients' own expectations, as they had anticipated a positive response from their doctor.

In the following extract Dr. Berta has noticed that Hilda has put on weight since her last visit in spite of being prescribed a diet at a previous visit. The initiation of this sequence is marked by a *QSI one* in line 47.

Example 19 Consultation N° 8 (Doctor: Berta, Patient: Hilda)

47 D: *¿Cómo es Uste– para comer grasa–?*
Do you usually eat fatty food?

48 P: *Eh: la verda– es que ahora yo me estoy cuidando y todo lo que es grasa lo he*
Eh: the truth is that I'm looking after myself now and

49 *dejado de la–o incluso cuando como pollo, al pollo se le saca el cuero se se*
I don't touch any fatty food. Even when I eat chicken, chicken I take the skin off

50 *come sin, sin el cuero y trato de evitar la grasa naturalmente.*
and I eat it without, without the skin. I try to avoid any fatty food obviously.

51 *Ahora si me pregunta si me gusta le digo que sí, pero no, no=*
Now if you ask me if I like it I'll tell you that I do, but no, no=

52 D: *=¿Y la fritura, el chancho, el cordero?*
=And fried food, pork, lamb?

53 P: *No, cordero no consumo, chancho muy a lo lejo–=*
No, I don't eat lamb, pork rarely=

54 D: *=¿Chuleta?*
=Chops?

55 P: *Muy a lo lejo–, muy a lo lejo–*
Very rarely, very rarely

56 ... *(N)*
... (N)

Dr. Berta does not offer any kind of feedback at any stage in this sequence. She seems to be interested only in checking whether the patient has been following a low-fat diet. This is reinforced in line 47, *¿Cómo es Uste– para comer grasa–?* ("Do you usually eat fatty food?") and in line 52, *¿Y la fritura, el chancho, el cordero?* ("And fried food, pork, lamb?"). The doctor's choice of high-lipid food items in her questions could even be interpreted as an indirect reprimand, or the food items as markers to express doubt as to whether the patient has in fact been following the prescribed diet. In line 56 there is a period of silence. From the noises heard on the recording, the doctor was probably writing in the patient's file.

The conversation continues when Hilda breaks the silence by expressing her concern about her weight gain. Here the patient's initiation of talk while the doctor has left a pause contradicts the finding of Heath (1992), who suggests that doctors' speech style modulates patient participation and that note-taking can work to silence the patient. Thus, in the above example we might have expected the patient to feel uneasy about making a further contribution to the speech. However, it is possible that Hilda interpreted Dr. Berta's prolonged non-interaction as a form of reproach and felt the need to restore *face* in the event by breaking the silence.

Example 20 Consultation Nº 8 (Doctor: Berta, Patient: Hilda)

57 P: *Lo que má– me preocupa es el peso doctora la obesida–. Hoy día me pesaron*
What concerns me most is my weight, doctor, the obesity. Today I've been weighed

58 *yo juré, he jurado que todo este tiempo que no la he visto me he, he como se*
I swore, I swear that for the whole time since I last saw you I've, how can

59 *llama me he cuidado he deja–o la carne roja, he estado comiendo*
I say it, I've been looking after myself, I haven't touched red meat, I've been eating

60 *prácticamente pollo, pescado. Juraba que había baja–o y: y:=*
mainly chicken, fish. I'd swear I would have lost weight and=

Once again the doctor does not respond to the patient's concern. (We may say here that Dr. Berta displays no shift in *footing*). Rather, she continues questioning her patient about her eating habits and in so doing maintains her alignment to the *Doctor voice* that seeks further information from her patient.

Example 21 Consultation Nº 8 (Doctor: Berta, Patient: Hilda)

61 D: *=¿Y pan?*
=And bread?

62 P: *Muy poco pan*
Very little bread

63 D: *¿Cuánto po'?*
How much?

64 P: *Uno al día*
One a day

65 D: *¿De qué tipo de pan ... marraque[ta ha]llulla?*
What kind of bread? Marraque[ta ha]llulla?

66 P: *[No, no] estoy comiendo centeno o del otro*
[No, no] I'm eating a low-calorie bread, or the other

67 *con fibra ¿cómo se llama? ... integral*
one with fibre, what's it called? ... wholemeal.

This time Dr. Berta focuses on Hilda's bread consumption and uses an elliptical form to suggest a sense of urgency: *¿Y pan?* ("And bread?"), *¿Cuánto po'?* ("How much?"), *¿De qué tipo de pan?* ("What kind of bread"?), even though Hilda appears to show an awareness of the kind and amount of food to be eaten while on a low-fat diet (*Muy poco pan*, "Very little bread"; *estoy comiendo centeno*, "I'm eating a low-calorie bread"), and responds in the negative to the doctor's questions relating to foods high in fat such as fried food, pork, and lamb chops. Dr. Berta appears not to offer her patient any support or understanding when she says she is making an effort to lose weight; on the contrary, she takes the patient's actual weight (as weighed by the assistant nurse before the consultation) as proof of lack of compliance, and makes a negative comment in this regard:

Example 22 Consultation N° 8 (Doctor: Berta, Patient: Hilda)

68 D: *Ya, pero igual digamo– ha pasado un mes desde que la vi*
O.K., but (you've put on weight in any case). It's a month

69 *la semana la vez pasada=*
last week since I saw you=

The first minimal feedback – *Ya* ("O.K.") – is uttered in line 68, but this is followed by the conjunction *pero* ("but") which contradicts the patient's own account of her dietary intake. While the weight gain is a bio-medical fact, Dr. Berta is quick to dismiss Hilda's claims that she has been complying with the dietary recommendations. An alternative stance for the physician could have been to investigate further why the diet is not working at the bio-medical level, as well as to consider whether any socio-relational factors may account for Hilda's apparent inability to follow her prescribed diet.

In contrast to this scenario, the data includes other interviews where a more sympathetic approach is in evidence. In the following transcript the patient has not complied with the recommendation that she should measure her blood pressure regularly, but the doctor adopts affiliation rather than reproach as his discourse strategy:

Example 23 Consultation Nº 21 (Doctor: Daniel, Patient: Yolanda)

91 D: *¿Se ha controlado la presión pa' ver cómo ha anda–o?*
Have you checked your blood pressure to see how you've been doing?

92 P: *Eh: no fíjese*
Eh: not really

93 D: *No . . . vamo– a ver*
No . . . let's see

Dr. Daniel initiates the dialogue with a *QSI one* in line 91, which seeks to establish both a blood-pressure reading and the patient's compliance. The difference between this example and the previous one is that Dr. Daniel uses the mirroring *No* ("No") in line 93 to confirm the patient's last utterance and then follows this with an offer to check the patient's blood pressure on the spot.

Example 24 takes up the same theme, the checking of blood pressure, so it is interesting to compare the two. Gina has also failed to comply with her doctor's request to measure her blood pressure regularly. However, unlike Dr. Daniel, Dr. Berta does not use the admission of non-compliance as a cue to perform the blood-pressure test. Instead, she remains silent.

Example 24 Consultation Nº 7 (Doctor: Berta, Patient: Gina)

11 D: *[¿Se ha seguido] tomando la presión Uste– en su casa?*
[Have you been] taking your blood pressure at home?

12 P: *No, no me la he seguido tomando, doctora*
No, no I haven't been taking it, doctor

13 D: . . . *(N)*
. . . (N)

. . .

51 . . . *Veamo– cómo está la presión ahora=*
. . . Let's have a look at you blood pressure now=

After the silence in line 13 Dr. Berta resumes the conversation by introducing the topics of smoking and diet. Then in line 51 she asks to check her patient's blood pressure.

A comparison of these two examples indicates the variable timing of consultation routines. Some doctors (as in Example 24) tend to favour a pattern of listing the medical issues first and then attending to medical procedures, while others (as in Example 23) may prefer to act on information provided by the patient, such as a statement of non-compliance, as it is reported.

In this section we have seen the different discourse strategies that doctors may use when making an evaluation of the patient's progress, and particularly when responding to non-compliant behaviour. Compliments, both direct and indirect (Examples 15, 16, 18), and encouragement (Example 23) contrast with reprimands implied through actual silence (Examples 19, 24), non-interaction with information the patient is providing (Examples 17, 19–21) or an implication that the patient is not being truthful (Example 22).

Cordella (in press), researching patient non-compliance within the framework of politeness theory, found that doctors used a variety of discourse strategies to deal with this behaviour, ranging from those that threaten the positive *face* of the patient to those that seek to maintain it. Dr. Daniel's response to Yolanda's non-compliance in Example 23 above (mirroring her utterance, offering to take her blood pressure) is an invitation to her to participate in a *face-saving act*, whereas doctors' non-engagement behaviour in Examples 17, 19–21, 22 and 24 (silence, unresponsiveness, implied criticism) could be understood as *face threatening* to their patients. Reprimand was one of the strategies used by all four doctors in the Cordella (in press) study. While not all of the examples in this section demonstrate doctor disapproval, it is interesting to note that those patients who had been non-compliant did not express any resistance to being reprimanded. Further, in all of the examples it was evident that the patient played a more passive role, and that the interaction of participants was essentially asymmetrical.

Table 10 shows that doctors' discourse favoured an evaluation of patients' test results or treatment over a discussion of patient compliance by a factor of

Table 10. Sub-functions of *Assesment and review*

Sub-function	**Frequency**	**%**
Assessment of test results or treatment	27	61.4
Assessment of patient compliance	17	38.6
TOTAL	44	100

roughly 3:2 (61.4 % : 38.6%). This may be because the purpose of the follow-up visit was specifically to discuss a set of test results the patient brought to the consultation or to check up on the efficacy of a previously prescribed treatment.

4.3 Alignment to authority

In this study, doctors' discourse was characterized by use of the Spanish pronominal system as a way of asserting authority in the consultation and alignment to the medical institution. These pronouns were explicitly uttered in the speech, although they could have been expressed as verb endings (Butt & Benjamin 1988). Specifically, three discourse strategies were identified, which aimed to give credibility to:

a. *The performance of self*, through use of the first-person singular *yo* ("I").
b. *The performance of self within the institution*, through use of the first-person plural *nosotros* ("we").
c. *The performance of other doctors*, through use of the third-person plural *ellos* ("they").

The following extract shows how Dr. Ana asserts her authority in the consultation by incorporating *yo* ("I") into her summary of the patient's previous visit:

Example 25 Consultation N° 1 (Doctor: Ana, Patient: Alicia)

168 D: *Yo recuer– bueno, la dejé con control, pero la idea era*
I remem– well, I left you for a check-up, but the idea was to

169 *mandarla a hacer algo así o psicoterapia*
ask you to do something like that or psychotherapy

The first-person singular in *Yo ... la dejé* ("I ... left you") here reinforces Dr. Ana's role as "I, the doctor, am in a position to ask you, the patient, to perform a specific action". The fact that the patient does not resist this linguistic performance of self indicates her willingness to co-operate in this asymmetrical framework of interaction.

Example 26 shows the use of *nosotros* ("we") that includes both the doctor who is talking as well as the medical establishment in which she works:

Example 26 Consultation Nº 5 (Doctor: Ana, Patient: Esteban)

40 D: ...*Sí, lo tratamos como una micosis=*
...Yes, we treated (the case) as a mycosis=

41 P: =<*WH Sí WH*>=
=<WH Yes WH>=

42 D: *=y lo dejamos con eh Fungium por diez día–*
=and we prescribed Fungium for you (to be taken) for ten days

We will recall this episode as the *Summary* of the patient's last visit in Example 11 above. Here the doctor's use of the first-person plural sets the medical treatment in the wider context of the hospital: *lo tratamos* ("we treated (you)"). It is as if the institution is the one responsible for the patient's well-being and not simply the doctor, as was the case in the previous example. Through pronominal emphasis Dr. Ana implies that her individual authority is strengthened by the collective authority of the hospital and that the two cannot really be differentiated. Of course, since the institution *per se* does not exist without the medical personnel to represent it, it could be argued that Dr. Ana is exploiting a false attribute on this occasion.

The next example shows how the doctor summarizes a diagnosis given by other doctors in the hospital. This is achieved by using a form of the third-person plural pronoun *ellos* ("they") to make the distinction between what the doctor recalls from the last visit and the diagnosis provided by the orthopaedic surgeon.

Example 27 Consultation Nº 13 (Doctor: Carlos, Patient: Olga)

12 D: ...*Nos vimos nosotros el 3 de octubre*... *había estado con un dolor*
...We saw each other on 3 October... you'd had a pain in your

13 *en la rodilla y en la muñeca derecha y en la muñeca derecha*
knee and right wrist, and in your right wrist

14 *le habían encontrado un túnel carpiano*
they'd found a carpal tunnel

This example differs from those of *performance of self* (*yo*) and *performance of self within the institution* (*nosotros*) since the speaker himself is fully excluded from the diagnosis he gives to the patient: *le habían encontrado* ("they'd found"). The doctor's task is simply to summarize and report the work of other specialists (in this case, the orthopaedic surgeon); his own credibility is not at issue. Nonetheless, the explicit utterance of the third-person plural pronoun by Dr. Carlos as a person of authority works to assert the authority of the other

Table 11. Discourse strategies used in *Alignment to authority*: summary

Discourse strategy	Frequency	%
Performance of self (“*yo*”)	22	40.8
Performance of self within the institution (“*nosotros*”)	23	42.6
Performance of other doctors (“*ellos*”)	9	16.6
TOTAL	54	100

health professionals who are responsible for the diagnosis, and his professional role as *animator* of their findings, in turn, reflects his own authority in the institution.

Table 11 summarizes the relative frequency with which each of these three discourse strategies occurred in the data, and shows that the authorizing pronouns “I” and “we” were used almost equally, and outweighed the third category “they” by a factor of 5:1. A closer examination of the patterns found across doctor–patient dyads in Table 12 reveals some interesting, if somewhat weak, trends that may indicate patient gender as a variable in the relative frequencies of these discourse strategies. All of the doctors who attended both female and male patients (Dr. Ana, Dr. Carlos, Dr. Daniel) used both *performance of self* and *performance of self within the institution* strategies more frequently (higher M values) with male patients than female patients (with the exception of Dr. Carlos, whose *performance of self* frequencies were reversed). Such preferential usage of “I” and “we” in the doctors’ discourse may be interpreted as a way of neutralizing the power position of male patients. While doctors have medical authority independent of their gender, males as such still occupy a privileged position in Chilean society (Yáñez 1999), and it would not be unexpected to find them asserting their social superiority in a medical consultation. These specific discourse strategies could be understood as an attempt on the part of doctors to avoid the potential for conflict between medical authority and male authority.

An interesting pattern also emerges in the analysis of *performance of other doctors*. Although this was the least frequently used strategy, only male doctors used it: Dr. Carlos used it exclusively with male patients, whereas Dr. Daniel used it exclusively with female patients. This may be due to the need for involvement of third parties in the management of the individual patient’s health problem (e.g. reference to a specialist or a medical technician), but may also say something about female doctors’ reluctance to neutralize their authority. This

Table 12. Discourse strategies used in *Alignment to authority*: frequencies for individual doctors and male/female patients

Discourse strategy	Dr. Ana		Dr. Berta	Dr. Carlos		Dr. Daniel		TOTAL
	F (n=3)	M (n=3)	F (n=3)	F (n=3)	M (n=3)	F (n=4)	M (n=3)	
Yo ("I")								
N	5	9	2	3	2	0	1	22
M	1.6	3.0	0.6	1.0	0.6	0.0	0.3	40.7%
Nosotros ("We")								
N	3	5	0	2	10	1	2	23
M	1.0	1.6	0.0	0.6	3.3	0.2	0.6	42.6%
Ellos ("They")								
N	0	0	0	0	7	2	0	9
M	0.0	0.0	0.0	0.0	2.3	0.5	0.0	16.7%
TOTAL	8	14	2	5	19	3	3	54 100%

is also reflected in the high frequency of usage of *Performance of self* among female doctors (M values ranging from 0.6 to 3.0) as compared with male doctors (M values ranging from 0.0 to 1.0). Further, in the two discourse strategies involving the institution overall, male doctors tended to show higher ranges (M = 0.0 to 3.3) compared to female doctors (0.0 to 1.6).

4.4 Summary

From Tables 8, 10 and 11 presented in this chapter, it can be seen that *Seeking information* was the function most frequently used by the *Doctor voice* in the follow-up consultations of this study, with 356 occurrences noted. Next was the *Alignment to authority*, with 54 recorded examples. The third function of the *Doctor voice*, *Assessment and review*, featured only 44 times. Table 13 summarizes the relative frequencies of these functions for individual doctors. *Seeking information* was not only the function most frequently used overall (78.4%), but also the most frequent in the discourse of all four doctors. Dr. Carlos recorded the highest value, with a relative frequency of 31.1. He also used the other two functions more frequently than the other three doctors (3.3 and 4.0). Dr. Ana shared with Dr. Carlos a liking for *Alignment to authority*, whereas both Dr. Berta and Dr. Daniel had little recourse to it, with mean findings of just 0.6 and 0.8 respectively.

Table 13. Functions of the *Doctor voice*: frequencies for individual doctors

Doctors	n	Seeking information		Assessment and review		Alignment to authority		Total
		N	M	N	M	N	M	
Dr. Ana	6	80	13.3	11	1.8	22	3.6	113
Dr. Berta	3	19	6.3	2	0.6	2	0.6	23
Dr. Carlos	6	187	31.1	20	3.3	24	4.0	231
Dr. Daniel	7	70	10	11	1.5	6	0.8	87
TOTAL		356	78.4%	44	9.7%	54	11.9%	454

4.5 Conclusion

In this chapter I have shown that there is a prevalent use of questions in the *Doctor voice*. I have also confirmed West's (1984) suggestion that *QSI chain* and *QSI multiple choice* strategies do not lead patients to answer fully with all the information required: part of the question remains unanswered because of the type of discourse form used to ask it.

It has also been shown that the *Doctor voice* includes the interpretation of the test results and the feedback that doctors give to patients when compliance is expected. This presented interesting discourse patterns ranging from silence (Example 19) to affiliative strategies (Example 23).

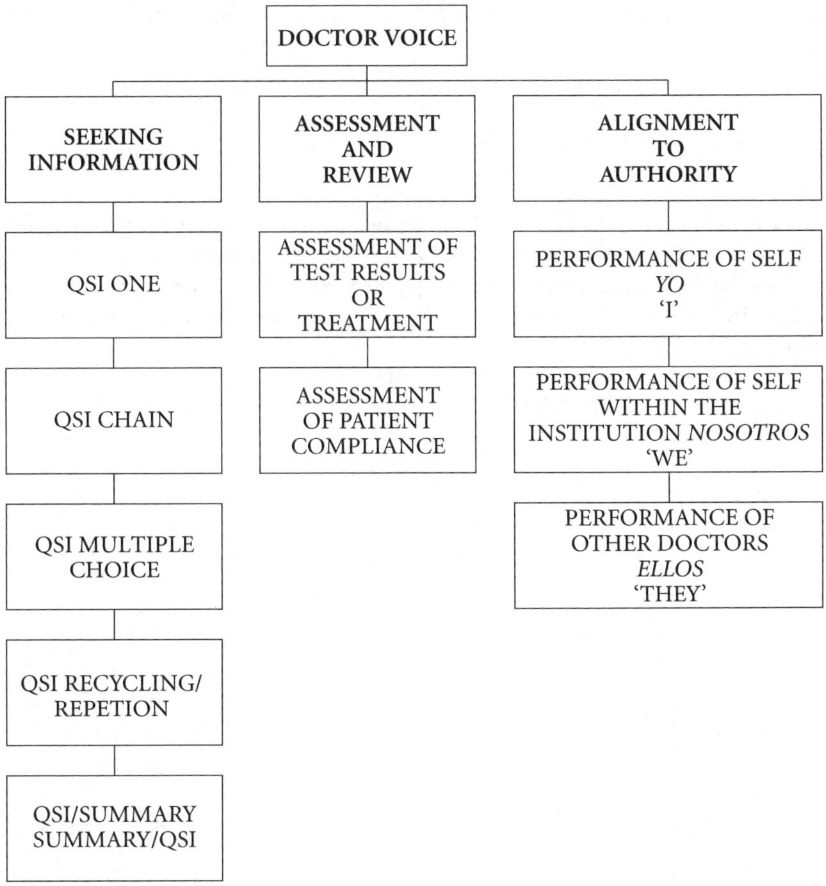

Figure 3. Discourse functions and strategies of *Doctor voice*

In terms of doctors' alignment to the medical institution it was possible to observe that the Spanish pronoun system can serve to express the stance that doctors take in the discourse. The use of the first-person pronoun *yo* ("I") reinforces the doctor's individual authority in the speech; the second-person plural form *nosotros* ("we") conveys that the individual doctor's authority is supported by the institution where the consultation takes place and by the medical profession at large; the third-person plural form *ellos* ("they") reports the findings or recommendations of other medical specialists in a way that both distances the speaker from any direct responsibility for the report while nonetheless implying an underlying colleagueship from which the patient is excluded.

Figure 3 illustrates the three main functions of the *Doctor voice*, each of which can be performed using a number of discourse strategies identified in this chapter.

Note

1. "It is still bullet-proof" is an example of the many metaphors drawn from the military that are in use in Chile. Although such metaphors have always been common in Chilean Spanish, the long years of military dictatorship in the '70s and '80s have increased the use of the lexicon in everyday talk. Military metaphors serve to make the "communication more colorful" (Smith 1997).

CHAPTER 5

The *Educator voice*

The *Educator* authors a *voice* of knowledge in the medical field that has been acquired through years of study and practice in the profession. This *voice* shares medical information with patients in order to help them better understand their health condition and appreciate the benefits of the recommended treatment. In so doing it aims to promote the principles of preventative medicine and encourage compliance. The *Educator voice* also works together with the *Doctor voice* in its alignment to medical practice.

The principal function of the *Educator voice* is that of *Communicating medical information*. It operates most particularly in the management and treatment routine of the consultation, and focuses on informing the patient of the various aspects of the presenting health problem, including physiological background, the nature of the condition, lifestyle issues, the purpose and requirements of tests and procedures, medication and management, and prognosis. *Communicating medical information* can be divided into three sub-functions, namely:

1. *Communicating medical facts*
2. *Responding to patient discomfort*
3. *Communicating medical treatment and management*

It is now proposed to examine each of these aspects of the *Educator*'s role in turn.

5.1 Communicating medical facts

Three different subject categories within the sub-function of *Communicating medical facts* have been identified in the course of this study. These are:

a. Information regarding available test results
b. Information regarding proposed tests
c. Information regarding the functioning of the human body

These categories are associated with the factual, scientific and medical knowledge that doctors share with their patients in order to allow them to become familiar with the medical aspects of their illness and treatment. (Some doctors prefer to withhold this information, and so deny the *Educator* a voice in the exchange. The possible reasons for and implications of this will be discussed in 5.7 below.) The *Educator voice* will be introduced through each of these three categories.

5.1.1 Information regarding available test results

In follow-up visits patients are required to bring the test results that were ordered at an earlier consultation. The interpretation of these results, as we saw in Chapter 4, is carried out through the discourse type *assessment of test results or treatment* that is conducted in the *Doctor voice*. At this point, doctors may also choose to provide their patients with additional, educational information to supplement the scientific data. This is accomplished through use of the *Educator voice*, in which the doctor is able to author a text based on his medical knowledge.

Example 28 Consultation N° 10 (Doctor: Carlos, Patient: Leonel)

56 D: *El antígeno prostático para ver cómo está funcionando la próstata está*
The prostatic antigen to see how the prostate is working, to see if it's

57 *funcionando O.K. ... El examen de sangre para ver como está el sodio,*
working O.K. ... The blood test [is] to see (the level of) sodium,

58 *el potasio que eso se puede alterar por los diurético– que estaba tomando ...*
potassium since they can change as a result of the diuretic you're taking ...

...

71 D: *El colesterol un pelo más alto de lo normal. Lo normal es hasta 200*
The cholesterol level is a fraction higher than normal. Normal is up to 200

72 *y tiene 202*
and yours is 202

...

104 D: *Lo otro que está un pelo alterado es la creatinina que eso ve*
The creatinine is the other (thing) that's changed a fraction. This looks

105 *la función del riñón*
at how the kidneys are working

Dr. Carlos, adopting the *Educator voice*, explains to Leonel what each of the tests has measured, describes the side-effects of the diuretic medication, and informs him what a normal level of cholesterol would be and how his own reading diverges from this.

Example 29 is a longer and more detailed explanation about the patient's chest X-ray. Whereas Example 28 showed the doctor imparting factual and statistical information (the normal range of sodium and cholesterol levels in the blood), here the doctor endeavours to teach the patient, rather than simply inform, by showing and explaining to her what can be seen on the film.

Example 29 Consultation N° 10 (Doctor: Carlos, Patient: Olga)

63 D: *En la radiografía se demuestran algunas cosas. Aquí a ver para verlo con*
The X-ray shows a few things. Here, let's see if we can look at them

64 *un poco más de calma, a ver cómo explicarle. Aquí están los cuerpos*
a little more calmly, let's see how I can explain it to you. Here are the

65 *vertebrales. ¿Ya? Y aquí hacia lo– lados se ven un poco aumentado su*
vertebrae of the spine O.K.? And here, towards the sides, you can see the space slightly enlarged

66 *espacio y ahí salen incluso así como a ver no se visualiza bien, pero hay*
and there they come out, even if you can't see it very well, but here there's

67 *un poquito un cachito que en la vista lateral imagínese aquí tenemos este*
a slight swelling, from the side view, imagine that here we have

68 *es el corazón y aquí tenemo– todo– lo– cuerpo– vertebrales y aquí se ve un*
this is the heart and here we have all the vertebrae, and here you can see

69 *espacio entre un cuerpo vertebral y otro hay un espacio que aquí está*
a space between one vertebra and another, and here's a space that's

70 *[el disco vertebral]*
[the vertebral disk]

71 P: *[Eso negro]*
[that black thing]

72 D: *Eso negro que no se ve nada ahí pero hay un disco gelatinoso que*
That black thing which you can't see anything of here, but there's a gelatinous disk

73 *mantiene el espacio que permite lo– movimientos*
that maintains the space which allows the movements (to take place)

74 *si Uste– se fija en este otro espacio la parte anterior hay*
If you look at this other space, the earlier part, it's

75 *como una cosa más blanca y el espacio está más apretado*
like a whiter object and the space is tighter

76 P: *Sí=*
Yes=

We can observe here how the *Educator voice* emerges in the discourse. In line 64 the instructional episode is initiated by *a ver cómo explicarle* ("let's see how I can explain it to you"), which establishes the participation framework of the consultation as one in which the doctor, having the medical knowledge, is able to educate the patient, who lacks the medical knowledge. Dr. Carlos shows the patient her chest X-ray and at the same time explains what can be observed in it. This is done by using the adverb of place *aquí* ("here"), followed by the verb *estar* ("to be") + body part, *aquí están los cuerpos vertebrales* ("here are the vertebrae of the spine"), *aquí está el disco vertebral* ("here's the vertebral disk"). This helps the patient to locate the vertebrae within the X-ray. Similarly, the *Educator voice* explains the extent to which the vertebrae are affected. The doctor says, *aquí hacia lo– lados se ven un poco aumentado su espacio y ahí salen ... un poquito un cachito* ("here, towards the sides, you can see the space slightly enlarged and there they come out ..."). The inclusion of the colloquial word *cachitos* ("slightly enlarged"), used in the diminutive form, may be an indication of the doctor's attempt to make his description easily understood by the patient. He also seems to be consciously avoiding medical jargon when he refers to the position of the vertebrae, and anatomical structures are expressed in lay terms: *aquí tenemos este es el corazón y aquí tenemo– todo– lo– cuerpo– vertebrales* ("... here we have this is the heart and here we have all the vertebrae") in line 68. In addition, Dr. Carlos captures Olga's attention and interest by involving her in the explanation: *imagínese* ("imagine") in line 67, and *si usted se fija* ("if you look") in line 74.

5.1.2 Information regarding proposed tests

The *Educator voice* can also be used to give an account of a medical procedure the doctor advises the patient to have. This is illustrated in Example 30. The patient suffers from diabetes, and has brought to the consultation the result of his glycaemia test, which indicates that the level of glucose in his blood is within normal parameters. The doctor would like to carry out another test to ascertain whether this level is maintained over a period of a month.

Example 30 Consultation N° 18 (Doctor: Daniel, Patient: Victor)

75 D: *...Eh: ... sí, me interesaría saber cómo, cómo sigue el régimen durante el*
...Eh ... yes, I would like to know how, how you follow your diet over

76 *mes, hay un examen que no es ese pa' chequearlo día a día, solamente*
a month, there's a test that isn't the one to check the level every day since

77 *da una fotografía de ese momento solamente, pero hay otro– que, que*
that one gives only a picture at a particular moment, but there's another

78 *evalúa má– o meno– como ha estado dentro del me–*
that checks roughly how you go over a month

The *Educator voice* begins with *hay un examen* ("there is a test") in line 76 and goes on to explain the purpose of the test the doctor would like to be undertaken, and how it differs from the test already carried out.

5.1.3 Information regarding the functioning of the human body

During the consultation, doctors may explain to their patients various biological functions of their bodies. This is presented in the following two extracts. In the first of these, Dr. Carlos ascribes a reason for Olga's back pain, while in the second he offers an explanation for the numbness in her arm.

Example 31 Consultation N° 13 (Doctor: Carlos, Patient: Olga)

75 D: *... el organismo reacciona frente a una situación de roce generando más hueso*
... the body produces more bone when there's friction

76 P: *Ya=*
O.K.=

77 D: *=Y esos cachitos despué– a la larga producen problemas aquí se ve más*
=and afterwards those small bumps in the long run produce more trouble. Here you can see

78 *acentuado aún llega hasta aquí afuera y eso va produciendo dolor en la espalda,*
the swelling is more accentuated, and even reaches the surface here, and this is what causes your back pain,

79 *pero eso no implica la molesia en el brazo*
but it doesn't explain the pain in your arm

In line 75 Dr. Carlos initiates the *Educator voice* with a general medical fact. Lines 77–78 expand on this, both by introducing further information and by gradually linking Olga's particular complaint to a broader understanding of the reasons for this failing of the human body. Line 78 draws all these threads together with the conclusion *eso va produciendo dolor en la espalda* ("and this is what causes your back pain"). The doctor has used the colloquial word *cachitos* ("small bumps") in line 77 instead of less familiar medical terminology (e.g. *protuberancia*, "protuberance"), in order that his patient can understand what he is saying – in other words, that the *Educator voice* is effective.

Thus far Dr. Carlos has given a general account of Olga's problem, and provided a contextual explanation for the back pain, but has not resolved why she is also experiencing numbness in her arm. The discourse marker *pero* ("but") in line 79 reveals and emphasizes (Carranza 1998: 56) that a further educative episode is needed. This occurs later on in the consultation, as follows:

Example 32 Consultation Nº 13 (Doctor: Carlos, Patient: Olga)

124 D: *Digamo– los huesitos que pasan por ahí o sea los huesitos que*
Let's say the tiny bones that pass through there, or rather the tiny bones that

125 *están ahí no dejan pasar fácilmente un nervio que queda atrapado entonces eso*
are there, don't allow the nerve to pass through easily, and so it gets trapped, which

126 *comprime un poco el nervio y eso produce este adormecimiento del*
compresses the nerve a little and causes the numbness in your

127 *bra[zo].*
a[rm].

The explanation for the numbness is given by using *entonces* ("so"), a marker of cause and effect, in line 125. The *Educator voice* helps Olga to understand her back pain and her arm numbness as physiological conditions. At the same time, this demonstration of the doctor's expertise parallels the alignment to medical authority that we saw earlier in the *Doctor voice*.

5.2 Responding to patient discomfort

In this study it was common for patients at follow-up visits to complain of symptoms related to their medical condition or to the side-effects of medication or treatment. These utterances prompted the doctor's *Educator voice* to explain the cause and nature of the symptoms to the patient and to account for the earlier decision to follow a particular treatment regime. The discourse forms used in the explanations varied.

One of my findings was that doctors frame patients' complaints as a medical issue for which they, and the medical institution in which they are employed, are solely responsible. As will be seen in the examples below, the *Educator voice* then defends any implication of medical mismanagement when responding to expressions of patient discomfort. There is a shift in footing away from the function of *communicating medical facts* towards a discourse that shows alignment to the medical institution and a belief that any decision taken by the institution is irreproachable. The three main characteristics of this phenomenon are:

a. Doctors frame patient discomfort as a medical issue that requires a medical interpretation
b. Doctors express complete faith in the medical decisions taken in previous consultations, affirming either directly or indirectly that these were the right decisions
c. Doctors minimize the side-effects associated with prescribed treatments

A set of examples will illustrate these three characteristics. In the first, Yolanda is a 70 year-old female patient who is visiting her doctor for a check-up. She has recently discontinued a medicine that she had been taking for over ten years, and is now experiencing some discomfort.

Example 33 Consultation Nº 21 (Doctor: Daniel, Patient: Yolanda)

167 D: ... *El cuerpo por un lado se acostumbra a tener un medicamento. Pudiera*
... On the one hand the body gets used to the medication. You might

168 *tener alguna– molestia– pasajera– que despué– del me– deberían pasar*
have some temporary discomfort that should pass in a month.

Note here the use of *pudiera* ("might have"), a subjunctive form of the verb *poder* ("can"), and *pasajera* ("temporary"), which serve to minimize the *molestia* ("discomfort") the patient is experiencing. Similarly, earlier in the same consultation Dr. Daniel plays down the possible side-effects of the new medication:

Example 34 Consultation Nº 21 (Doctor: Daniel, Patient: Yolanda)

161 D: ... *El hecho de haber estado tomando harto tiempo puede que al cambiar*
... The fact is that, when you change the medication or discontinue it after you've been taking it for a long time,

162 *ahora al dejarlo esto– quince día– primero el primer, primer me– sienta*
for the first fortnight, the first, first, first month you may feel

163 *alguna– molestia– extrañas– alguna cosa porque en el fondo tiene*
some discomfort, something strange, because basically you've been

164 *algún medicamento*
on medication.

Here the patient's symptoms are presented as *alguna– molestia– extrañas– alguna cosa* ("some discomfort, something strange"). The use of *alguna cosa* ("something") minimizes the level of discomfort by leaving vague how the *cosa* ("thing") is to be defined. Similarly, the symptoms are framed as something unusual and "strange". The time frame is stated as brief: *quince día–* ("fifteen days") or *primer mes* ("the first month").

In the second example the patient has been suffering from headaches as a result (he believes) of changing the dose of his blood-pressure medication. This example is particularly interesting because the doctor neither queries the earlier recommendation to change the dose nor accepts the suggestion that the medication may be responsible for the headaches. Rather, he deflects any criticism of his medical authority by questioning the patient's attitude towards taking the medication instead.

Example 35 Consultation Nº 10 (Doctor: Carlos, Patient: Leonel)

49 D: *Puede ser ah el problema que frente a cambio de medicamento, suele a*
Ah, the problem could be connected to the change of medication. Sometimes it

50 *veces ocurrir alguna– veces explicaciones por culpa de lo– medicamento–,*
happens that, sometimes there are explanations that blame the medication,

51 *pero también está el factor humano que uno piensa que a lo mejor el*
but there's also the human factor for one thinks that the

52 *medicamento me está haciendo algún problema=*
medication is probably causing the problem=

53 P: *=Sí, sí ...*
=Yes, yes ...

The doctor introduces his discourse with *puede ser ah el problema* ("the problem could be") – a statement of "possibility and plausibility" (Butt & Benjamin 1988: 227) – and continues with a cautious *suele a veces ocurrir* ("sometimes it happens") and *algunas veces* ("sometimes") to indicate his alignment with the orthodox medical view that headaches are not usually associated with the medication. By contrast, the discourse marker *pero* ("but") in line 51 is followed by the verb *estar* ("to be") in the indicative, *pero también está el factor humano* ("but there's also the human factor"), giving greater emphasis to his stated belief in the possibility of a psychosomatic reaction to the change of medication. Dr. Carlos appears not to consider an alternative possibility; namely, that the headaches could in fact be organic in origin and the physician (either Dr. Carlos himself or a colleague) who prescribed the medication made a mistake. We have to assume that, if the problem persists, the patient will be given a different dosage of the same medication, or a new prescription.

This leads us already to two important findings regarding the *Educator voice*. Firstly, that "education" is circumscribed to the doctor's own knowledge and personal views, which in turn are bound to and uphold the medical practices of the institution. Other knowledge or opinions – including the patient's own subjective reports – are not easily entertained. Secondly, and hand-in-hand with this, the *Educator voice* works not only to inform the patient of medical facts, but also to present information that will protect professional credibility. In our example, Dr. Carlos uses particular discourse strategies to promote his own explanation for Leonel's headaches. Had he not done so, and an admission of error been made, both he and the medical institution he represents would have *lost face* (Brown & Levinson 1987; Goffman 1967). Education and authority can thus be seen to align when the doctor's credibility is made vulnerable. Further examples of this behaviour will be encountered throughout this chapter.

In the third example the patient has been experiencing pain in his ankle. The doctor has not requested any tests, claiming that the "wait and see" approach is the best way of managing the problem.

Example 36 Consultation Nº 5 (Doctor: Ana, Patient: Esteban)

57 D: *Porque no había ningún elemento como para pensar en algo má–*
Because there was no reason to think otherwise

58 *Así que por eso que no yo me quedé tranquila y observar solamente porque*
That's why I remained calm and only observed because

59 *hay mucha, de repente uno tiene muchas molestia–*
there are many, sometimes one feels many discomforts

...

62 *Y se da cuenta que muchas van y pasan sola–*
And one realizes that many come and go by themselves

...

64 *Hay muchas molestias que son así y que no vale la pena en gastar en*
There are many discomforts like that, and it's not worth paying

65 *exámenes y cosa– así ...*
for tests and such like ...

67 *=Claro, uno la la la cuando hay algunas orientan a cierto tipo de cosas y*
=Of course, when some (discomfort) points to something specific, then

68 *ahí uno le pone má– ojo, pero:=*
you've got to take a closer look, but=

...

70 *En este caso era muy inespecífico, era una cosa que:=*
In this case it was unspecific, it was something that=

...

72 *Sin gusto a nada entonce– no no habla mucho como para tampoco*
Nothing was showing, nothing much could be said, so there was not much

73 *po' pa' asustarse=*
to be frightened about

Dr. Ana uses the *Educator voice* to convince her patient that he has no evident medical problem. She explains her decision not to have him undergo medical tests in line 57, *no había ningún elemento como para pensar en algo má–* ("there was no reason to think otherwise"), in line 70, *En este caso era muy inespecífico* ("In this case it was unspecific"), and in line 72, *Sin gusto a nada* ("Nothing was showing"). These utterances are also intended to stress that the doctor has made the right decision. The other utterances in Dr. Ana's talk are attempts at teaching the patient not to pay attention to every discomfort he experiences. Her view is that anyone can feel uncomfortable, so there is no need "to be frightened" or to be "paying for tests".

Although Dr. Ana says that discomfort can often be disregarded because it cannot be linked to anything in particular, she does mention that there are other kinds of discomfort (without specifying them) that could indicate a medical problem. When this occurs, *ahí uno le pone má– ojo* ("you've got to take a closer look"). In this way the *Educator voice* implies that the doctor has a superior ability to distinguish between these unspecified symptoms and the patient's current discomfort, and to treat them both with the necessary expertise.

5.3 Summary

The analysis found that the discourse strategies of the *Educator voice* varied, depending on whether the doctor was communicating medical facts or responding to accounts of patient discomfort. In the former, and particularly evident when discussing the functioning of the human body (5.1.3), the doctor's factual explanations were part of a learned and rehearsed medical speech, a lecture drawing on acquired medical knowledge. When responding to accounts of patient discomfort (5.2), on the other hand, the *Educator voice* functioned in two distinctive types of discourse. In the first, doctors again projected themselves as both *author* and *principal*, in Goffman's (1981) sense, of a rehearsed medical speech; in the second, however, they sought to construct their professional credibility and to fend off any challenge to their authority. Credibility may be at issue when there is a possibility that the patient's symptoms are a direct consequence of inappropriate medical management. The study found that doctors tended to undermine (by ignoring) any suggestion of an association between discomfort and prescribed treatment by stressing the probability that the patient's symptoms were most likely psychosomatic or the result of the patient's own behaviour. This issue is discussed further in Chapter 9.

5.4 Communicating medical treatment and management

Doctors will sometimes discuss with their patients the medical treatment or management they recommend. This is because the third sub-function of the *Educator voice* imposes on the patient certain requirements to act in ways they may find undesirable (e.g. to take medication, have an operation, lose weight, stop smoking, etc.). The doctor's advice may even be openly contested in certain circumstances (Fisher & Todd 1986a). As shown in the examples above, diagnostic medical information or responses to discomfort were never challenged in the consultations recorded in this study. Discussion of medical treatment and management, however, is a dynamic and potentially negotiable discourse, and one that unfolds throughout the interview. In this section I analyse the discourse strategies available to the *Educator voice* to outline the proposed course of treatment and to achieve a mutually agreeable outcome.

The starting-point for the analysis was to identify the discourse strategies involved in the function of giving advice. Sometimes doctors may express the opinion that a certain course of treatment is an absolute necessity and that there is no other option: I will call this strategy a *marker of inevitability*. At other times doctors may leave open the possibility of an alternative course of treatment: this strategy is designated a *marker of conditional inevitability* and its utterances are expressed in the conditional mood. In the analysis that follows, these two types of Spanish markers are examined using passages from the transcripts. This is followed by an exploration of a third discourse strategy, use of the impersonal pronoun *uno* ("one") in doctors' speech. Finally, some passages in which doctors and patients negotiate the medical treatment and management are analysed.

5.4.1 Spanish markers of inevitability

The *marker of inevitability* directs in its discourse structure that the instruction of the speaker be followed. In my study, one of the common markers of inevitability was the construction *hay que* + infinitive ("one must"). Prieto-Castillo (1999) classifies *hay que* as a discourse strategy that denotes *despersonalización* ("de-personalization") of the act. In other words, the subject is not explicitly mentioned in the speech. He writes:

> *[En] este recurso [lingüístico], cuyo paradigma está dado por ... el empleo del verbo "haber", llega a tener la fuerza que reconocimos a la universalización. En realidad, se trata de una suerte de universalización por la acción. Las expresiones se alzan también como leyes, como mandatos para cumplir ... Cada una de esas afirmaciones aparece como si nadie la hubiera dicho, como un valor en sí mismo.* (1999: 114)

> [In] this [linguistic] tool whose paradigm is given ... the use of the verb "to have to" comes to have the force of being recognized as a universal. In reality, it is universal because of the action it accomplishes. The utterances are also raised as laws, orders to be followed ... Each of these affirmative statements appears as if nobody had said them, as if they had a value in themselves.

Other markers of inevitability recorded in the data were:

a. The verb structure *ir* ("to go") in the 2nd person singular + *necesitar* ("you will need to")
b. The verb structure *ir* ("to go") in the 2nd person singular + *requerir* ("you will be required")
c. The verb structure *ir* ("to go") in the 2nd person singular + *a tener que* ("you will have to") (Salazar 1978)

All of these constructions carry a non-optional, or obligatory force, as though the doctor were *animator* of a speech whose *author* and *principal* were some unnamed higher authority. They are always presented as statements in the imperative mood.

The following examples of *markers of inevitability* highlight the presence of one particular type of marker. The first of these presents a patient who had articulated feeling lonely and lacking in energy, and who reported that she did not spend time with her sister when she came to visit her, which created a difficult situation for both of them. The doctor tries to encourage her patient to interact with other people and gives her advice as to what she should do when her sister visits.

Example 37 Consultation N° 3 (Doctor: Ana, Patient: Carmen)

232 D: *Entonce– va a tener que: eh: e– difícil ¿uhm?, pero va a tener que tratar de*
So you'll have to: eh: it's difficult, uhm? But you will have to try to

233 *hacerse como un día que vaya ella y olvidarse de to-o lo otro y*
to make it a day just for her and forget everything else

234 *sentarse má– a conversar, ya porque Uste- tiene la idea que ella va como pa'*
relax and have a chat because you have the impression that she comes, as it were,

235 *cumplir ¿ya?:=*
out of obligation O.K.?=

In this passage Dr. Ana uses a *marker of inevitability* in line 232 (*va a tener que*, "you will have to") followed by the verb *tratar* ("try"), which softens the effect of the obligation, presumably to increase the likelihood of Carmen accepting the advice. The *Educator voice* here states that the patient would benefit from company, and that she needs to spend time with her sister when she comes to see her.

The next example illustrates the use of the marker *hay que* ("one must") in the discourse. Here the patient is suffering from stress and high blood pressure. The doctor uses her *Educator voice* to explain that the medication needs to be changed and the stress level reduced.

Example 38 Consultation N° 4 (Doctor: Ana, Patient: David)

254 D: *Lamentablemente, como por lo que me cuenta va a necesitar má– dosi–*
Unfortunately, from what you're telling me you'll need to increase the dose,

255 *o agregar un poquito má– de medicamento de por ese lado ¿Ya?. Eh*
or increase slightly your medication. O.K.?

256 *en la cosa de la presión... se exacerban con la tensión o sea hay que manejar*
In regards to your blood pressure ... it gets worse with stress, so it means that one must manage

257 *la tensión.*
the stress.

Dr. Ana's aim here is to educate David that there is a correlation between his high blood pressure and stress level. This is achieved in line 256 by explaing that high blood pressure *se exacerban con la tensión* ("gets worse with stress"), and that, therefore, *hay que manejar la tensión* ("one must manage the stress"). She insists on this point again later in the discourse, as follows:

Example 39 Consultation Nº 4 (Doctor: Ana, Patient: David)

262 D: *Hay que atacar principalmente la cosa nerviosa es lo principal que hay*
One must mainly attack the nerve problem, that's the main

263 *que manejar*
thing that one must manage

Dr. Ana reiterates the importance of reducing David's level of stress by repeating *hay que* ("one must") in line 262, accompanied by two synonymous verbs *atacar* ("to attack", i.e. overcome, control) and *manejar* ("manage"); by using the adverb *principalmente* ("mainly"); and by the noun phrase *lo principal* ("the main thing"). Clearly the repetition is designed to reinforce the importance of the doctor's advice.

5.4.2 Spanish markers of conditional inevitability

The imposition (Brown & Levinson 1987) of the *marker of conditional inevitability*, by contrast, is less forceful because it functions in the conditional mood. When giving advice to their patients, doctors in the study often expressed this using the conditional form of the verb *ser* ("to be") – *sería* ("it would be"). Example 40 demonstrates this usage. The patient suffers from obesity, and her doctor is advising her on how to manage her weight.

Example 40 Consultation Nº 8 (Doctor: Berta, Patient: Hilda)

72 D: *... lo ideal sería que... Uste– se comprara una pesa, una buena pesa, una*
the ideal thing would be ... for you to buy scales, good scales,

73 *buena balanza ...*
a good weighing scales ...

...

90 *lo ideal sería digamo– que anotara en un papelito*
the ideal thing would be, say, to write down your weight.

Later in the consultation Dr. Berta advises Hilda to keep a record of her weight. The use of the *marker of conditional inevitability* in line 72 (*lo ideal sería que*, "the ideal thing would be") could be interpreted as an acknowledgment by the doctor that purchasing the scales may be an imposition on the patient. By the same reasoning, the conditional marker *lo ideal sería* ("the ideal thing would be") in line 90 may convey an empathy with the burden this places on the patient.

Functional usage of the Spanish *marker of inevitability* and *marker of conditional inevitability* found in this study suggests that doctors are able to modulate their discourse from a more to a less forceful recommendation. This notion is consistent with previous studies (Davis 1988; Todd & Fisher 1993; van Dijk 1995b, 1996, 1997b; Wodak 1996, 1997, 1999b) which found that those who are in a position of power have available different discourse strategies to achieve desired ends. In certain circumstances, a recommendation in the conditional mood may be more persuasive: in Example 40 above, the doctor's use of the conditional *sería* is more polite than its imperative form and may potentially encourage greater compliance. Further, by being presented with the option to accomplish specific tasks (to buy scales and keep a record of her weight), the patient is handed some personal power for managing her own health; this allows us to recognize the use of the conditional mood to perform a *face-saving act*, which again may foster compliance. This idea also is further explored in Chapter 9.

5.4.3 The impersonal pronoun

The impersonal pronoun *uno* ("one") was also recorded in doctors' speech in the routine of communicating medical treatment and management. We have already encountered instances of this in Examples 35 and 36 above: *uno piensa que a lo mejor el medicamento me está haciendo algún problema* ("one thinks that the medication is probably causing the problem") in lines 51–52 and *uno tiene muchas molestia* ("one feels many discomforts") in line 59 respectively. In these utterances *uno* may be understood to represent the generic plural "patients" or the noun phrase "many patients I see". Example 41 provides a further passage for analysis.

Example 41 Consultation Nº 3 (Doctor: Ana, Patient: Carmen)

205 D: ... *uno necesita de un, de un cierto apoyo social de amigo–* ...
... one needs a kind of social support, of friends ...

...

227 D: ... *uno requiere de otra– persona–, amiga–, no sé qué sé yo a juntarse al*
... one needs other people, a friend, to get together in some way in

228 *(El) Club de Tango o Centro de Madre lo que sea, lo que sea, pero necesita*
(The) Tango Club or Mothers' Centre, whatever it may be, but you need

229 *un grupo eso es inevitable ¿ya? Uno necesita algo donde poder hablar*
a group, that's essential. O.K.? One needs a place where one can talk,

230 *ademá– que ahí uno se da cuenta ademá– de otra– realidade– ve la– cosa–*
for there's another way of looking at things

231 *como distinta también la visión de, de otra– persona–*
another way of looking at things

Here Dr. Ana uses the *Educator voice* to stress the importance of the patient forming part of a social group and having a network of friends with whom to exchange thoughts and feelings. The sentiment *uno necesita ... un cierto apoyo social de amigo–* ("one needs a kind of social support, of ... friends") in line 205 is reinforced in line 227, *uno requiere de otra– persona–, amiga–* ("one needs other people, a friend"). The doctor also suggests specific venues where Carmen might find friends. Even though the choice of a social group is left to the patient, *lo que sea* ("whatever it may be"), the doctor presents it as a necessary step (*inevitable*) in line 229 if the patient is to feel less isolated and lonely, and goes on to explain why it is important for her to meet other people.

By citing examples of the social activities that are available to the patient, the *Educator voice* highlights socio-cultural aspects of Chilean society as well as socio-cultural expectations placed on women to belong to an approved gender-specific group. *Uno* here can be understood as "Chilean women in your socio-cultural situation". The doctor's choice of *uno* over *nosotros* ("we") also reinforces the different socio-demographic background of the participants. Whereas Dr. Ana made frequent use of *nosotros* to align her performance to the institution (cf. Table 12), she does not align herself to the patient; instead, *uno* in this case creates a distance between doctor and patient. The impersonal pronoun has the implied sense of "Chilean women in your socio-cultural situation (not mine)".

A second, contrasting function of *uno* was also identified in the study. In Spanish, *uno* "is similar to the English 'one' in that it is often an oblique way of saying 'I' or 'we'" (Butt & Benjamin 1988: 307). Thus, sometimes self-reference is intended. In Example 42 below, *uno* in lines 94 and 98 refers to the doctor herself and to the institution she represents.

Example 42 Consultation Nº 4 (Doctor: Ana, Patient: David)

92 D: *Yo encuentro que Adax es una buena opción para Uste– el, el Adax ¿ya?*
I believe that Adax is a good option for you, Adax O.K.? Yes

93 *si vamos a tener le voy hacer un cambio en las dosis pero vamos a tener*
we'll need, I'll need to make a change in the dose but we'll need to

94 *que por lo meno mantenerlo por lo meno durante un tiempo: y uno lo que*
maintain it, at least for some time. What one often does is

95 *hace mucha– vece– bajando dosi– y haciendo cambio para no tenerlo por tanto tiempo::*
to (start) decreasing the dosage and changing it in order not to stay (on the medication) for a long time

...

98 D: *=Claro en general uno lo deja por un tiempo: limitado pero, Uste–*
=Of course one usually leaves it for a time, a limited time, but you need

99 *necesita má– dosi– uhm necesita má– una ayuda má–*
a larger dose uhm you need more help, more.

In both lines 94 and 98 the doctor uses her *Educator voice* to inform the patient how the medication is usually administered. In this way the patient acquires relevant medical information. What is interesting here is that the use of *uno* conceals the agent of the information. The impersonal pronoun conveys the idea that Dr. Ana is simply voicing and applying a set of rules established *as the norm* rather than making her own personal recommendation for treatment. *Uno* is stronger than the plural form *nosotros* ("we") that we explored in 4.3 in establishing a higher authority for the doctor's proposed management and treament. While *nosotros* sought to align the individual doctor with his/her institution and profession, *uno* implies that the recommendation goes beyond even these and corresponds to the *universalización* ("universal") identified by Prieto-Castillo above.

We can observe that the doctor's discourse in this passage displays both a change of *voice* and a shift of footing, from the *Doctor voice* (with the enunciated first-person pronoun that was examined in 4.3) of *Yo encuentro* ("I believe") in line 92 to the *Educator voice* (with the impersonal *uno*) in line 94. Had Dr. Ana continued with the first-person pronoun *yo* ("I", as in *yo lo que hago mucha– vece–*) instead of using *uno* ("one"–*uno lo que hace mucha– vece–*), her own recommended treatment and management would not have been contextualized as part of standard medical practice.

5.4.4 Persuasive education

Earlier in this chapter the sub-function of *Communicating medical treatment and management* was described as occurring within a potentially negotiable discourse. Whereas *Communicating medical facts* and *Responding to patient discomfort* placed the patient in a largely passive role as *recipient* of medical information, this third sub-function of the *Educator voice* may be thought to offer some scope for patients to act as *participants* in the process of choosing appropriate treatment and management of their health problem. The examples in this section reveal whether or not this occurs in practice, and analyses the discourse strategies used by doctors to encourage a particular outcome.

In the following extract the patient is suffering from depression. The doctor advises psychotherapy sessions, which she claims will be very helpful.

Example 43 Consultation Nº 3 (Doctor: Ana, Patient: Carmen)

101 D: ...*A ver, bueno el ánimo está mejor aunque todavía claro,*
... Let's see, well, you're feeling better, although it's still clear

102 *queda cosa. Yo, yo le hablé alguna ve– que sería bueno en alguna–*
there's something wrong. I, I've sometimes told you that it would be good in

103 *ocasione– apoyo con en psicología o con psicoterapia*
some instances to have some psychological or psychotherapy support

She starts by summarizing the patient's state in the continuous present. Carmen is in better spirits, *el ánimo está mejor*, although there are still some remnants of depression, *queda cosa* ("there's something wrong"). This factual observation provides a platform for giving her advice using a *marker of conditional inevitability*: *sería bueno* ("it would be good"). It is understood that the phrase *en alguna– ocasione–* ("in some instances") refers to the present moment and to Carmen in particular, and that it is she who will benefit from therapy. Dr. Ana's discourse strategy is thus to give positive feedback to the patient in the present tense, followed by a qualifying statement, and finally a suggestion for treatment using a *marker of conditional inevitability*. This sequence smooths the way for introducing the idea of psychological help, and may be more likely to persuade the patient to accept the doctor's advice.

In the following passage from the same visit, however, Carmen explains that she is employed (*yo trabajo*, "I work") in line 105, and is worried that her daily routine will be affected by the doctor's proposed therapy.

Example 44 Consultation Nº 3 (Doctor: Ana, Patient: Carmen)

104 P: *Sí, sí lo que pasa doctora que yo: estoy dejando mi salud un poquitito de*
Yes, yes what's been happening, doctor, is – let's say – I've been neglecting my health a little.

105 *lado digamo– para lo– permiso– es decir como yo trabajo tengo que viajar es decir*
As for sick leave, since I work I've got to commute and that means taking

106 *a a mi significa toda la mañana eh: acá, entonce– sí tengo que pedir, no sé*
taking up the whole morning, so if I need to ask (for sick leave) I don't know

107 *¿cuánto tiempo eh: cita a esto, si e– una ve– al me– una ve– a la semana o:?=*
how often it is once a month, once a week or?=

108 D: *=Es como generalemte es como una o cada una o cada do– semana– ah en general*
=It's usually once a week, or every fortnight

Carmen expresses her concern that the therapy will conflict with her work commitments and raises the issue as a potential obstacle to complying with Dr. Ana's advice. The discussion continues below, with Carmen stating that her decision to attend psychotherapy sessions depends on her employer: *lo quiero conversar con mi jefe* ("I want to talk it over with my employer") in line 111. This is because sick leave has to be granted every time she goes to psychotherapy, which would be every week or every fortnight, as Dr. Ana has indicated.

Example 45 Consultation Nº 3 (Doctor: Ana, Patient: Carmen)

110 P: *Eh: yo ni siquiera me averigué tengo en todo caso la hojita que Uste– me dio,*
Eh I didn't even make enquiries. In any case, I've got the note you gave me,

111 *pero: lo quiero conversar con mi jefe para, pero:: no he podido conversar porque*
but I want to talk it over with my employer but I haven't been able to talk to him because

112 *pasa en [reunione–]*
he's has been in [meetings]

113 D: *[Claro]*
[Right]

Dr. Ana does not comment on Carmen's concern about her work obligations, but in lines 114–118 below simply reiterates her belief that the treatment she has proposed would be valuable:

Example 46 Consultation Nº 3 (Doctor: Ana, Patient: Carmen)

114 D: *=Claro sería bien bueno porque por lo meno– la parte de la, de la*
=Of course it would be very good because at least in regards to your

115 *angustia, de la ansieda– hay cosa– que lo– remedio– ayudan, pero también*
apprehension, your anxiety, there's a remedy, something that helps, but it also

116 *depende mucho como la persona enfrente la situación y en eso ayuda*
depends a lot on how the person faces the situation, and in this respect

117 *harto la psicotera:pia=*
psychotherapy is very helpful=

118 P: *=Me imagino que sí*
=I imagine so

Once again the doctor's discourse includes a *marker of conditional inevitability*, *sería bien bueno* ("it would be very good") in line 114. This time it is emphasized by the adverb of manner *bien* ("very") and by *claro* ("of course") that initiates the passage. The proposition that medication is not the only answer to the patient's problem is also introduced. This is indicated by the use of the conjunction *pero* ("but"), which links the medication to the psychotherapy, co-constructing them as complementary treatments in lines 115–117. The patient latches onto the doctor's talk with the concurring *me imagino que sí* ("I imagine so") in line 118.

Dr. Ana makes one final utterance on the subject, which is shown in this last example from the consultation.

Example 47 Consultation Nº 3 (Doctor: Ana, Patient: Carmen)

119 D: *¿Ya? Así que yo creo que Uste– se ayudaría así es que la idea que*
O.K.? So I think you would benefit, so the idea is that when you see

120 *cuando Uste– vea que se pueda hacer el hueco ojalá, lo pueda hacer ¿ya?*
that you can manage to make the time, hopefully you'll do it. O.K.?

121 *Para Uste– sería bien beneficioso ¿ya?*
It would benefit you greatly. O.K.?

The phrase *así que yo creo* ("so I think") in line 119, with its assertive use of *yo* ("I") in the *Doctor voice*, indicates that Dr. Ana has now decided that the patient will attend psychotherapy sessions. This is then softened with the following *marker of conditional inevitability*, *se ayudaría* ("you would benefit"), and with the subordinator of time, *cuando* ("when"), which indicates that the doctor has in fact taken into account the patient's alleged lack of time. The discourse continues with *ojalá* ("hopefully") and *para Uste– sería beneficioso* ("it would benefit you greatly"), both of them intended to reassure the patient who needs this kind of treatment.

Examples 43–47 demonstrate how the doctor utilizes various discourse strategies to persuade her patient to comply with the medical recommendation. The *Educator voice* explains what is necessary, and why, and adopts conditional markers to ease the patient towards acceptance of a treatment that confronts her current lifestyle. The patient's work commitments are finally acknowledged in lines 119–120. Line 119 steers the discussion briskly towards acceptance of the treatment as a *fait accompli* and allows Dr. Ana to conclude the episode in the *Doctor voice* of authority.

The next example demonstrates how the *Educator voice* can be used to help patients acquire an understanding of medical procedures and then influence their decisions about treatment. Olga has been suffering from pain in her arm. She has visited an orthopaedic surgeon who advised her to have an operation, and is now consulting her family doctor, where she brings up her fears about the operation. Dr. Carlos explains to her why the surgery is desirable:

Example 48 Consultation Nº 13 (Doctor: Carlos, Patient: Olga)

136 P: *... si uno, y si uno no se opera ¿qué pasa?*
... if one doesn't have an operation, what will happen?

137 D: *siente las molestias que Uste– percibe eso [podría ir empeorando]*
You'll feel the discomfort you're feeling now [It could get worse]

138 P: *[Por eso si no me opero] estar más relajada*
[But if I don't have] an operation I should be less stressed

139 D: *No, no, no*
No, no, no

140 P: *Me gusta jardinear por ejemplo*
I like gardening, for example

141 D: *Pero Uste– va a notar las limitaciones Uste– debe ir aceptando sus*
But you'll notice the limitations. You'll have to accept your

142 *limitaciones en el fondo si se opera lo más probable que ocurra es que*
limitations. If you have the operation, what's almost certain is that

143 *eso vaya a recuperarse en forma optima y Uste– va a poder hacer su vida*
you'll recover perfectly well and you'll be able to carry out your life

144 *completamente normal=*
in a completely normal way=

145 P: *=Ya=*
=O.K.=

146 D: *=Si no se opera debe aceptar un poco esas limitaciones que frente a*
=If you don't have the operation, you'll have to accept limitations to your

147 *movimientos manuales, siente limitaciones siente adormecimiento,*
hand movements, you'll feel limitations, numbness,

148 *dolore– nocturno– que a veces se despierta por esas molestias y hay*
night pain that will sometimes wake you up. There are

149 *alguno– tratamiento médico que pueden tratar de combatir eso=*
some medical treatments to fight that=

150 P: *=Ya=*
=O.K.=

151 D: *=Pero no son tan espectaculares como lo de la cirugía, la cirugía*
=But they're not as spectacular as surgery.

152 *le han explicado que es algo rápido=*
they've explained to you that surgery's quite quick=

Olga initiates the episode by expressing her concern about the operation (*si uno, y si uno no se opera ¿qué pasa?*, "if one doesn't have an operation, what will happen?") in line 136. She fears that the pain will interfere with her usual activities, such as gardening (line 140). Although framed as a statement (*Me gusta jardinear*, "I like gardening"), this utterance is an implied question: Olga is trying to ascertain the extent to which her life will change if she does not have the operation. In lines 138 and 139 both participants understand and frame the medical problem differently. This disruptive event is an example of what

Wodak (1996: 2) describes as a *frame conflict* (see Section 2.3, "Everyday and institutional talk"). The patient believes that her problem is associated with her stress (*si no me opero estar más relajada*, "if I don't have an operation I should be less stressed" in line 138), whereas the doctor (who has claimed earlier in the discourse that her problem is linked to a hereditary malformation of the bones in her arm) sees a physiological explanation and responds to this notion in the negative (line 139).

Dr. Carlos's attitude towards the operation is expressed in the *Educator voice*. Education and persuasion work closely together in this episode to make the patient accept a decision made by the medical body (the doctor himself and the specialist who has examined the patient). On the one hand, a negative outcome is predicted if the operation does not go ahead. This is encapsulated in line 146, *si no se opera debe aceptar … limitaciones* ("if you don't have the operation you'll have to accept … limitations"): the discourse form of conditional clause followed by a *marker of inevitability* spells out to the patient that she will be responsible for her ongoing physical symptoms if she decides against the operation. This includes the possibility that her condition might worsen if the operation is deferred (*podría ir empeorando*, "it could get worse" at line 137), using the construction *podría* (conditional) + *ir* (infinitive) + gerund to convey progressive deterioration. On the other hand, the doctor's discourse strategies maximize the chances of success and predict a rapid recovery, using the positive adverbial phrases *en forma optima* ("perfectly well"), *completamente normal* ("completely normal") and *algo rápido* ("quite quick") in lines 143, 144 and 152 to appeal to a patient who fears not being able to carry out her usual activities. Surgery is not only desirable, it is *espectacular*!

The *Educator voice* in this example encourages patient compliance by presenting all the information that favours the operation and none that might show it in a less positive light. Alternatives to surgery are presented in an entirely negative way. Analysis of the discourse reveals that the *voice* of the *Educator* works with the *Doctor voice* in that the selection and presentation of information is performed in such a way as to reinforce the doctor's authority in the exchange. With this passage, our discussion of the discourse involving Leonel's headaches (Example 35 above) may be clearly recalled.

The data also included an example of the *Educator voice* disrupting (Wodak 1996) its own normal educator role. In Examples 49 and 50 the doctor reacts strongly to his patient's suggestion that she may be open to opinions beside his own when it comes to making a decision about her operation. The narrative is a continuation of the consultation that we encountered in Example 48 above.

Example 49 Consultation Nº 13 (Doctor: Carlos, Patient: Olga)

175 P: *. . . con algunas personas que han tenido este problema*
. . . some people who've had the same problem (have said to me)

176 *no te opere– que es horrible y fuera de eso al final uno queda igual=*
don't have the operation, for it's horrible and, besides, it made no difference in the end=

Dr. Carlos does not acknowledge that Olga is reiterating the fear she had already expressed in lines 138 and 140 (Example 48). Instead he proceeds with a somewhat didactic speech on the difference between professional and non-professional opinions.

Example 50 Consultation Nº 13 (Doctor: Carlos, Patient: Olga)

179 D: *¿Quién son médico–?*
Are they doctors?

180 P: *Eh, eh persona– paciente–=*
Eh, eh people, patients=

181 D: *=Exacto pero son pac[iente–]*
=Alright, but they're pat[ients]

182 P: *[Claro]*
[Of course]

. . .

206 D: *. . . No le pediría la opinión a otra persona que no sea especialista en el*
. . . I wouldn't ask the opinion of someone who's not a professional in the

207 *tema no creo que es buena fuente=*
field. I don't think that person would be a good source of information=

208 P: *=Ya=*
=O.K.=

209 D: *=De confianza*
=A Trustworthy (source)

210 P: <@@>=
<@ @>=

211 D: *=Ya yo no le estoy preguntando lo que tengo que hacer en un problema legal a un vecino*
=I don't ask my neighbour what I should do in a legal matter if he's

212 *si no es abogado=*
not a lawyer=

213 P: =<@*Ya*@>=
=<@O.K.@>=

214 D: =*Entonces uno tiene que ir donde gente que tenga experiencia porque*
=So one should go to those people who have (professional) experience because

215 *es re fácil opinar uh no te opere– con eso uno queda tranquilo porque dice lo*
it's very easy to give opinions: don't have an operation and you'll be right.

216 *que yo pensaba pero a lo mejor com– decirle a una persona*
It's like me telling a person

217 *que tiene una apendicitis uh no te opere– el no operarse*
who has appendicitis uh, don't have the operation. The failure to operate would

218 *significa la muerte probablemente para esa persona entonce– el caso no es*
probably mean death for that person, so it's not a matter of

219 *llegar y a lo que le digan si hacer es una fuente no muy=*
listening to what other people say if they're a source that is not very

220 P: =*No muy con[fiable]*
=Not very [trustworthy]

221 D: *[entendi]da entendida en el tema*
[knowledge]able in the matter

In this passage the doctor uses the *marker of inevitability*, *tiene que* ("have to/one should") in line 214 to stress that a suitable recommendation can only be made by a professional in the field. The opinions of those who are unqualified are not to be trusted (lines 206–207, 209). This observation is illustrated with the example of consulting a lay person about a legal matter (lines 211–212). Following this in line 214, an utterance commencing with a discourse marker of cause and effect, *Entonces* ("So") + an impersonal agent + *tiene que* repeats the idea that only someone with professional experience should be consulted for reliable information. Dr. Carlos also disregards the opinions of those people who have experienced the operation themselves. He then introduces a second example to reinforce his point, this time a case of appendicitis, and dramatizes the connection between failure to operate and *muerte* ("death"). This account can be interpreted as a strategy to persuade Olga to accept his advice by instilling fear, even though there has been no indication that conservative management of her arm pain could have fatal consequences. The cause-and-effect marker *entonces* ("so") is then repeated in line 218, which announces a repetition of the earlier statement in lines 206–207 that the opinion of those without medical authority have no validity.

Dr. Carlos continues along the same lines, in the form of advice to his patient, as set out in this last extract:

Example 51 Consultation Nº 13 (Doctor: Ana, Patient: Olga)

221 D: ... *Aquí en Chile lamentablemente somo– todo– potenciale– médico– y*
... Unfortunately, here in Chile we are all potential doctors

222 *todo– damo– consejo– Mire la vecina se tomó esta pastillita, tiene lo mismo tuyo*
we all give advice look, my neighbour took this medicine, and she had the same problem as you.

223 *De ahí partimo– con un error ¿Tendrá lo mismo? Pero esta pastillita*
This is the start of the mistake. I wonder if she has the same problem? But this medicine

224 *le hizo bien pero a lo mejor esta otra persona no tenía lo mismo y esa*
made her better, but, at best, that person may not have had the same

225 *pastillita además le hace daño, pero todo el mundo está recetando así hay que*
problem. Moreover, it may damage her, and yet everyone is giving prescriptions,

226 *tener cuidado un poco en ese sentido ...*
so you have to be a little careful in this sense ...

Throughout this episode the doctor aligns himself to the institution by rejecting any medical opinion or advice given by non-professionals, even though he couches his utterances in an inclusive way by using the plural forms *somo–* ("we are") and *damo–* ("we give") in lines 221 and 222, and reinforces this idea again in line 225: *todo el mundo está recetando* ("everyone is giving prescriptions"). *Aquí en Chile* ("here in Chile") offers a socio-cultural explanation for Olga's "misconception" that she might find it helpful to listen to the advice of her friends or neighbours. Since the doctor rejects this cultural attitude, he warns her against it, using the cause-and-effect marker, *así (que)* ("so"), followed by the warning *hay que tener cuidado* ("you have to be careful") in line 226. The implication is that patients should not venture beyond their boundaries: by moving into medical territory where they do not belong they risk "damage" (*daño*). Only by being *cuidado[so]* ("careful") – that is, by complying with the doctor's recommendation – will they receive safe and appropriate treatment.

5.5 Summary

I have shown that the *Educator voice* draws on a different set of discourse strategies when engaged in the routine of communicating medical treatment and management. These include the *marker of inevitability* (e.g. *tiene que/debe*, "to have to", *hay que*, "one must"), which places an obligation on the patient to follow the doctor's instructions; the *marker of conditional inevitability* (e.g. *sería bueno*, "it would be helpful"), which stresses the desirability of following the doctor's instructions; and the impersonal pronoun *uno* ("one"), which may be used to align the doctor to a higher authority (Example 42) or to emphasize the different social status of doctor and patient (Example 41).

From the analysis in this section it can be seen that, for doctors, these discourse strategies are resources to minimize the negotiating power of their patients. In other words, doctors adopt a more sophisticated discourse when the communication routine is one in which their control ought potentially be more flexible. The *Educator voice* not only imparts information for the benefit of the patient, but also "disrupts" its educator role when the patient presents alternatives or challenges to its authority. As these positions threaten the doctor's *face*, the *Educator voice* will remind the patient, either gently or rather less subtly, of their respective institutional roles as a *face-saving act*. It is noteworthy that the doctor's intentions for the patient's management and treatment were always achieved in the examples given above.

Figure 4 provides a summary of the discourse functions and strategies of the *Educator voice*.

5.6 Statistical findings

In this chapter I have identified the different subject categories of the *Educator voice* in the communication routine of management and treatment at follow-up visits. The relative frequencies of these categories are presented in Tables 14 and 15. Of the 22 consultations studied, 15 featured the *Educator voice* engaged in communicating medical facts, responding to patient discomfort, or explaining treatment and management. Seven consultations (32% of the total), however, lacked any instructional episode in the discourse. Tables 14 and 15 therefore show findings only for the 15 consultations in which the *Educator voice* was present.

More than half of the episodes featuring the *Educator voice* were found to involve communicating medical treatment and management to the patient

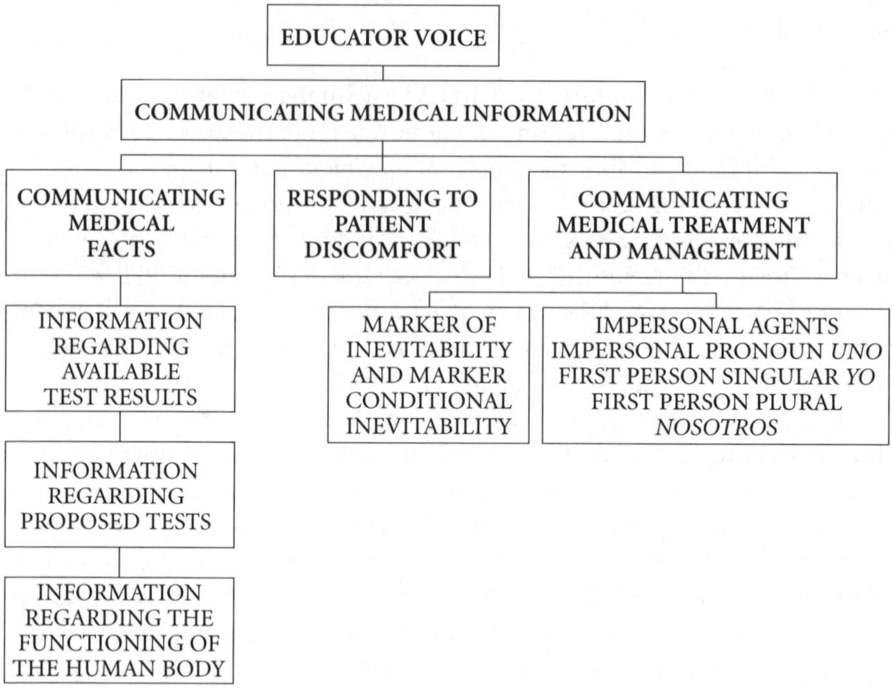

Figure 4. Discourse functions and strategies of *Educator voice*

(56.8%). At the other end of the scale, patients were given information about proposed or recommended tests (such as we saw in Example 30 above) on only 4 occasions. These findings are summarized in Table 14. Table 15 further divides the data for the 15 consultations into usage patterns of the four doctors in the study. The most striking finding in this Table is the far higher incidence of education regarding medical treatment and management by the two female doctors (M = 9.5 and M = 3.3 respectively). However, although Dr.

Table 14. Functions of the *Educator voice*: summary

Subject category	Frequency	%
Available test results	22	16.7%
Proposed test results	4	3.0%
Functioning of the human body	16	12.1%
Patient discomfort	15	11.4%
Medical treatment & management	75	56.8%
TOTAL	132	100%

Table 15. Functions of the *Educator voice*: frequencies for individual doctors

Doctor	n	Available test results		Proposed tests		Functioning of the human body		Patient discomfort		Medical treatment & management		Total
		N	M	N	M	N	M	N	M	N	M	
Dr. Ana	6	10	1.6	3	0.5	4	0.6	6	1.0	57	9.5	80
Dr. Berta	3	1	0.3	0	0	0	0	0	0	10	3.3	11
Dr. Carlos	6	10	1.6	0	0	11*	1.8	7	1.1	8	1.3	36
Dr. Daniel	7	1	0.1	1	0.1	1	0.1	2	0.2	0	0	5
TOTAL		22	16.7%	4	3.0%	16	12.1%	15	11.4%	75	56.8%	132

n = number of consultations
N = frequency
M = mean frequency per consultation
* These were initiated following requests from patients

Berta outscored her male counterparts in this one category, she showed a very limited usage of the *Educator voice* overall. Dr. Daniel did not communicate medical treatment and management information on even one occasion, and his performance was low in the other subject categories as well. Dr. Ana was the only doctor of the four to communicate information on every subject, followed by Dr. Carlos who discussed all the categories with his patients except for that of proposed tests. Thus, while the *Educator voice* was found to favour female doctors when it came to discussing with patients the "hows and whys" of managing their health condition, in other respects it was not shown to be gender-specific.

Table 16 explores this idea further by examining whether the gender of the patient may influence the use of the *Educator voice*. Here Dr. Ana is found to have provided her male patients more information across the board. The results for Dr. Carlos show the opposite trend: he is far more forthcoming with his female patients when it comes to giving an account of how the body functions (10:1) or explaining treatment and management (7:1). Within the limitations of his very low scores, Dr. Daniel shows a weak preference for communicating information to his female patients.

These gender-based differences may have multiple explanations. For example, Dr. Ana's results may be connected with the relative frequency with which men and women attend medical consultations. As we saw in Chapter 3, men visit their doctor on average three times less often than women. Male patients who seldom visit a doctor may therefore receive more information at each consultation than female patients who visit more regularly. In the case of Dr. Carlos, it may be that he is responding to the greater number of queries from female patients (see Chapter 7, "Patients' voices"). It is also worth noting that those male patients who received most information were professionals (an engineer and a publicist), whereas the one who received the least was the employee of a hardware store. While the doctor's perception of the patient's ability to comprehend medical information may be a factor in providing education, it was also found in this study that the two professionals received almost twice the consultation time as the non-professional. A similar pattern was described in Waitzkin's (1985) study, which found a correlation between patients' education, social class, length of visit and the amount of information given in the consultation. It is possible that better educated patients are more assertive in asking questions that prompt a reply by the *Educator voice* and therefore extend the length of the appointment. The age variable appears not to be related in this instance, since the male employee was in his mid-50s, the same as that of the publicist, while the engineer was in his mid-30s.

Table 16. Functions of the *Educator voice*: frequencies for individual doctors and male/female patients

Category	Dr. Ana		Dr. Berta	Dr. Carlos		Dr. Daniel		Total
	F (n=3)	M (n=3)	F (n=3)	F (n=3)	M (n=3)	F (n=4)	M (n=3)	
Available test results								
N	2	8	1	5	5	1	0	22
M	0.6	2.6	0.3	1.6	1.6	0.2	0.0	16.7%
Proposed tests								
N	0	3	0	0	0	0	1	4
M	0.0	1.0	0.0	0.0	0.0	0.0	0.3	3.0%
Functioning of the human body								
N	0	4	0	10	1	1	0	16
M	0.0	1.3	0.0	3.3	0.3	0.2	0.0	12.1%
Patient discomfort								
N	1	5	0	4	3	2	0	15
M	0.3	1.6	0.0	1.3	1.0	0.5	0.0	11.4%
Medical treatment & management								
N	19	38	10	7	1	0	0	75
M	6.3	12.6	3.3	2.3	0.3	0.0	0.0	56.8%
TOTAL	22	58	11	26	10	4	1	132

n = number of consultations
N = frequency
M = mean frequency per consultation

5.7 Absence of the *Educator voice*

At the beginning of the previous section it was observed that the *Educator voice* was absent from 7 out of the 22 consultations recorded for this study. This finding prompts a number of questions. Are we to understand the absence of the *Educator voice* from those consultations as depriving the seven patients of the opportunity to acquire a better understanding of their health condition? Will this limit their chances of looking after themselves adequately? Is the absence of patient education in almost one-third of consultations contradictory to the basic teaching principles of the institution where the study was conducted? If we accept that the silencing of the *Educator voice* may be a problem, then what is its cause, and how should it be interpreted?

We have by now established that the relationship between doctor and patient is inherently unequal and that both the *Doctor* and *Educator voices* reflect and reinforce the asymmetrical frame. The doctor possesses and dispenses medical information, and the patient receives and complies with this information. The primary purpose of the *Educator voice* is to help the patient understand and follow the appropriate treatment and management for the presenting health condition through its principal function of communicating medical function. However, we have also seen that the *Educator voice* has a secondary function of asserting the doctor as the voice of authority and medical expertise in the exchange. When the patient challenges the doctor's recommendation (as we saw in Examples 50 and 51 above), the *Educator voice* may be rapidly invoked to remind the patient that this trespass into medical territory is unwelcome and inappropriate. At the back of the doctor's mind may be a concern that a knowledgeable patient will prove less tractable, will challenge the doctor's control over the consultation, and will pose a threat to the (jealously guarded) exclusivity of the medical establishment. This point will be further developed from a macro perspective of doctor–patient communication in Chapter 9.

Secondly, it was shown in Table 15 that 8 of Dr. Carlos's 11 instructional episodes regarding the workings of the human body were triggered by a patient asking a question. This suggests that those seven consultations that did not include the *Educator voice* may have been with patients who were reluctant to ask questions of their doctor.

5.8 Conclusion

The *Doctor voice* seeks information about the patient's current health condition, assesses patient compliance, and reads test results. The *Educator voice* then emerges in the discourse to explain these findings to the patient and to engage in further discussion in order to reach an acceptable regimen for ongoing management and treatment. The doctor's desired outcome is achieved with specific discourse strategies, including *markers of inevitability* and *markers of conditional inevitability*, which persuade the patient to comply with the medical recommendation. Both *Doctor voice* and *Educator voice* work together to maintain the doctor's control in the exchange, and the educational episodes are prescribed to information which reinforces and protects the doctor's professional credibility and alignment to the institution.

A third *voice* identified in doctors' speech remains to be examined, however, and this *voice*, unlike the other two, presents discourse features which are likely to be found in everyday conversations. The next chapter introduces the *Fellow Human voice*.

Chapter 6

The *Fellow Human voice*

During the consultation the doctor may converse with the patient using neither the *Doctor voice* nor the *Educator voice*, but a third *voice* which I have called the *Fellow Human voice*. The *Fellow Human* does not seek information about medical symptoms, tests or compliance (*Doctor voice*) and does not aim to educate the patient about the presenting health problem and its management (*Educator voice*). Rather, the function of the *Fellow Human voice* is to show empathy, and to encourage patients to tell their stories. In keeping with a holistic approach to medicine, which recognizes that a person's condition can sometimes be understood by looking at social factors that affect health – for example, ongoing problems in the family or workplace – the *Fellow Human* complements the *Doctor* and *Educator voices* in exploring the whole picture of the patient as a way of understanding the health problem. This chapter will investigate the discourse strategies that doctors use to invite their patients to open up about their personal situations and feelings, and to convey affiliation, interest and involvement. The *Fellow Human voice* engages in a discourse that is less *medically* (asymmetrically) framed than the *Doctor* or *Educator voices*, and is therefore important for a full understanding of the doctor–patient relationship.

This study has identified five functions of the *Fellow Human voice*. Doctors use this *voice* to:

a. Facilitate the telling of patients' stories
b. Assist the telling of patients' stories
c. Create empathy with the patient
d. Show special attentiveness to patients' stories
e. Ask questions unrelated to the patient's health

These five functions are characterized by a range of discourse strategies that will be illustrated in the following sections.

6.1 Facilitating the telling of patients' stories

In the data, doctors were shown to make use of three *continuer markers* (CMs) as prompts for patients to develop their stories. Following the conversation analysis of Jefferson (1979), Sacks et al. (1974) and Jefferson et al. (1977), Jurafsky et al. define a CM as a "short utterance which plays discourse-structuring roles" (1998: 2). The utterance usually occurs in a two-part sequence: in the consultative setting, the doctor's CM represents the first part of the sequence and the patient's response to it the second part. A CM cannot initiate a discourse by itself, needing the presence of a previous utterance. The function of the doctor's CM is to invite the patient to participate in the speech.

While the invitee may choose to accept or reject this invitation (Jefferson 1979: 80), very few patients in this study refused the opportunity to take the floor (1.1%, 3/261). In those situations, the doctor quickly regained control of the discourse. There was also one consultation in which the patient simply stated that she had nothing further to say, rejecting outright the opportunity given to her to elaborate on her remarks. In all other cases (98.9%, 258/261), patients were willing to take up the offer. Having noted those few instances of rejection, our attention will now focus on the discourse strategies used to encourage the patient's involvement.

Ya ("Yeah/O.K."), *Mm/Uhm* ("Mm") and *Mm/Uhm ya* ("Mm yeah/O.K.") were identified as the three CMs favoured by doctors. Stivers and Heritage (2001) describe "Mm, hm" as a way of conveying the listener's willingness to play the role of recipient of the story, but these CMs may also have a more interactive meaning attached to them. In some instances they can be interpreted as "I understand" and/or "I'm listening". In the following example, the patient is talking about the medication he has been taking and the doctor uses *Ya* ("Yeah/O.K.") to encourage him to continue.

Example 52 Consultation Nº 6 (Doctor: Ana, Patient: Flavio)

93 P: *El Flu– es la verda– que la última: semana parece que tomé una ve– o sea no*
The Flu– it's true that last week I seem to have taken it once a day, but I've

94 *me acordaba si ¿tenía que tomar lo– de la caja?*
forgotten whether I had to take those from the package

95 D: *El flu– el Fluxo me dice ¿Uste–?*
You say you're taking the Flu– the Fluxo?

96 P: *Sí*
Yeah

97 D: *Ya*
Yeah

98 P: *Ya así do– o tre– día– que no no lo– he toma–o*
Yeah, I haven't been taking it for two or three days

99 D: *Ya*
Yeah

100 P: *Pero: Eh: la verda– que durante el tiempo que me lo tomé=*
But: Eh: really during the time I was taking it=

Both the confirmation of the name of the medicine in line 96 and the patient's admission that he has stopped taking it in line 98 are followed by the doctor's *Ya* ("Yeah/O.K.") in lines 97 and 99. These utterances may be understood as *receipt markers*, which imply "I understand what you are telling me", "I'm listening to what you are telling me", or a combination of both. There is no evidence that use of this CM serves to quash the patient's contribution, since in both cases there is socio-cultural recognition that it has communicative intent (Gumperz 1982b) aimed at facilitating rather than disrupting the patient's talk.

The number of CMs used during a consultation appears to be dependent on the individual doctor's interest in having the patient take his/her turn to open up the narrative. This study has found some examples where only one CM was offered, severely restricting the patient's potential contribution to the discourse. On the other hand, several conversations were recorded in which the use of three or four CMs allowed patients to recount their story over an extended period of time. This differs markedly from the stereotypical medical exchange, in which a limited question–answer sequence is the normal pattern.

The following two examples are particularly interesting, as they contrast the number of CMs employed by a doctor in two different episodes of the same conversation. In the first there is recurrent use of CMs. This helps the patient to explain her symptoms in more detail and gives the doctor a fuller picture of the illness as it affects her patient's lifestyle.

Example 53 Consultation Nº 1 (Doctor: Ana, Patient: Alicia)

37 D: *Cuénteme en ¿qué situaciones ha presenta–o má– angustia?*
Tell me, in which circumstances have you experienced an increase in anxiety?

38 P: *En qué situacione–, por ser ahora han disminui–o la– angustia–*
In which circumstances, for now (I feel) they've diminished

39 D: *Ya:*
Yeah:

40 P: *Pero cuando <X X> una leve angustia fue cuando hubieron viento– o lluvia– muy fuerte*
But <X X> (I experienced) a small anxiety attack when it was windy or when it rained heavily

42 D: *Uhm ya*
Mm yeah

43 P: *Eh: resulta que estaba estudiando. Yo estoy estudiando ahora*
Eh: the fact is that I was studying. I'm studying now

44 D: *Ya:*
Yeah:

45 P: *Y: y me dieron sensacione– de salir arrancando de ir pa' mi casa y llegar a mi casa*
And: and I had this feeling to dash out and rush back home

46 *pero así de una pata–a*
in a flash

47 D: *Ya:*
Yeah:

48 P: *Lo único que quería era correr al lado de mi casa, dentro de mi casa:=*
The only thing I wanted to do was to run round my house, inside my house:=

In this earlier part of the consultation Dr. Ana uses her *Fellow Human voice* to encourage Alicia to remember one particular day when she experienced an anxiety attack. *Ya* ("Yeah/O.K.") is produced softly, and the elongation of the vowel *a* at the end of the CM *Ya* (in lines 39, 44 and 47) conveys that she is giving her full attention to the story and attempting to understand the event that created Alicia's distress.

Later there is only limited use of the CM in the discourse, which can be seen to restrict the patient's participation.

Example 54 Consultation Nº 1 (Doctor: Ana, Patient: Alicia)

80 D: ... *¿Cómo anda el ánimo?*
... How are you feeling?

81 P: *El ánimo ha andado bien*
I've been alright

82 D: *Ya*
Yeah/O.K.

83 P: *Ha andado bien y: de repente un poquito de angustia, pero superable, o sea ratito, es lo*
I've been alright. Sometimes (I feel) a bit of anxious, but I can overcome this,

supero al momentáneo, por rato– chico–
or rather, I overcome it for a while, it's temporary, for a short time

85 D: *¿Y cómo está durmiendo?*
And how have you been sleeping?

Here Dr. Ana uses the CM *Ya* ("Yeah/O.K.") in line 82 to invite her patient to take the floor, and Alicia then opens up about how she is handling her anxiety. In line 85, however, the patient's narrative is interrupted, as Dr. Ana does not follow with a further CM but resumes her questioning in the *Doctor voice*. This abrupt shift of footing effectively terminates the patient's account of her anxiety episode.

From these two examples we can observe that there is a direct relationship between the number of CMs uttered by the doctor and the number of opportunities patients are given to develop their narrative. The more CMs uttered by the doctor, the more potential chances there are for one of the patient's *voices* to come into play. In an ideal setting, doctors would utilize CMs frequently in order to encourage a more balanced framework of participation and to obtain the most comprehensive knowledge of the patient's condition. In practice, however, the use of CMs varies greatly. Time constraints in closely scheduled appointments are one factor, though, as we have seen, opportunities for patient participation are facilitated or limited largely at the doctor's discretion.

It is important to note that while this analysis shows the importance of CMs in medical consultations in Chilean Spanish, in other language/social groups the presence or absence of CMs may have different consequences. For example, it is conceivable that in other societies doctors' non-intervention in the speech could serve as a stimulus, rather than act as a deterrent to the patient's contribution. This would be contrary to the trend found in the present study.

Table 17 shows *Ya* ("Yeah/O.K.") as clearly the continuer marker most frequently encountered in the study, with a frequency of 81.2%. The other two

Table 17. Discourse strategies used in *Facilitating patients' stories*

Continuer marker	Frequency	%
Ya	212	81.2
Mm/Uhm	22	8.4
Mm/Uhm ya	27	10.4
TOTAL	261	100

CMs were used to a much more limited extent. Nevertheless, all three have the same purpose of furthering the patient's account.

6.2 Assisting the telling of patients' stories

The doctor may show an affiliation with the patient by collaborating in the patient's talk; this collaborative aspect of the *Fellow Human voice* is achieved through the *joint production* of speech. The ways in which two speakers perform a single proposition have been investigated by Falk (1980), Lerner (1991) and Schegloff (1984), among others. Joint productions differ from interruptions in that no attempt is made by one party or the other to re-take the floor.

The examples found in this study are consistent with Ferrara's description of joint productions, which discounts the view that these are to be understood as a "talk intruding into the talk of another" (Zimmerman & West 1975), or as a sign of violation of the conversational rules of speaking.

> Joint productions ... are a second speaker's attempt to contribute to the syntactic and semantic intent of the first speaker. At times joint productions are explicable as efforts to clarify, to ensure completeness or correctness in terms of information and truth value and these semantic wishes are performed with syntactically compatible contributions by a second speaker to the first speakers' utterance. The result is one sentence contributed by two interlocutors.
> (Ferrara 1992: 219)

Ferrara's description of joint production is consistent with Tannen's (1983) and Cordella's (1996) understanding of *co-operative overlap*, through which the building up of the discourse creates affiliation and camaraderie between participants (Coates 1996, 1998; Schiffrin 1984). In her 1992 paper, Ferrara enumerates four types of joint production:

a. *Utterance extension* – "the feasibility that a sentence or sentence analog [see Levinson 1983: 18] can be extended by a second speaker beyond the point at which the first speaker considered it complete necessitates discourse analysis of all utterances in tandem with the subsequent utterance(s) to determine if they are in fact complete at the first possible completion point or receive continuation by another" (217–218).

b. *Predictable utterance completion* – "speakers project their intended utterances well before their point of completion" (219).

c. *Helpful utterance completion* – "minimal additions offered by a listener who detects some difficulty on the part of a speaker in accessing an item in the mental lexicon" (220).

d. *Invited utterance completion* – "induced by initial speaker's eliciting the sentence completion from the second speaker by means of a word stretch (syllable elongation) followed by a brief pause" (221).

Analysis of the data in the present study has identified 24 occurrences of joint production of the patient's speech. The majority of these (68%, 17/25) belong to the first type, *utterance extension*. Some examples are given below.

6.2.1 Utterance extension

In her consultation with Dr. Carlos, Paola is talking about her breathing problems and the difficulties she experiences when taking a deep breath.

Example 55 Consultation Nº 14 (Doctor: Carlos, Patient: Paola)

101 D: *¿No puede respirar profundo?*
You can't take a deep breath?

102 P: *No siempre. Ahora sí=*
Not always. Now I can=

103 D: *=Ya=*
=Yeah=

104 P: *=Pero no constante de repente yo me trato de observar como es mi respiración=*
= But not always. Sometimes I try to observe what my breathing's like=

106 D: *=Ya=*
=Yeah=

107 P: *=Y no siempre llego*
= And I don't always fully inhale

108 D: *Hasta el fondo*
(To) the very end

109 P: *Entonces pienso ...*
So I think ...

We can observe from this passage that both doctor and patient are co-operating to build up the discourse. They do this by contributing one turn each in lines 107–108, so that the first utterance is complemented with a new one that expands upon it. The collaborative joint production is initiated after Paola's turn in line 107, *Y no siempre llego* ("And I don't always fully inhale"), which is followed by Dr. Carlos's *utterance extension* in line 108 *Hasta el fondo* ("(To) the very end"). Paola then continues in line 109 with *Entonces pienso ...* ("So I think ..."), indicating that she has not interpreted Dr. Carlos's *utterance extension* in line 108 as an intrusion on her speech, or an attempt to take control of the discourse, but rather as helpful encouragement for her to further the narrative. This discourse strategy is illustrated also in the following example:

Example 56 Consultation Nº 1 (Doctor: Ana, Patient: Alicia)

45 P: *Y: y me dieron sensacione– de salir arrancando de ir pa' mi casa y llegar a mi casa*
And: and I had this feeling to dash out and rush back home

46 *pero así de una pata–a*
in a flash

47 D: *Ya:*
Yeah:

48 P: *Lo único que quería era correr al lado de mi casa, dentro de mi casa:=*
The only thing I wanted to do was to run around my house, inside my house:=

49 D: *=Como má– protegi–a*
= To feel more secure

50 P: *Claro*
Of course

The patient describes her feeling of fear in line 48, which the doctor takes up in line 49 with the *utterance extension Como má– protegi–a* ("To feel more secure"). By engaging in this type of joint production, and making her own contribution, Dr. Ana conveys empathy with Alicia's account of her anxiety and fragility. If she had disagreed with the doctor's interpretation of her feelings in line 49, Alicia would have not replied with the agreement form *Claro* ("Of course") in line 50.

6.2.2 Predictable utterance completion

Only four examples of *predictable utterance completion* were found in the data. One of these can be observed in the following extract, in which the patient explains that his stress and the resulting insomnia have led to his taking sedatives again.

Example 57 Consultation Nº 1 (Doctor: Ana, Patient: David)

115 D: *¿Cuénteme Uste– tomaba me dijo que tomaba ante el Adax y el*
Tell me, you were taking, you told me that you were previously taking Adax and

116 *Bromasepán Uste– había tomado por año– había estado toma[ndo?]*
Bromasepán. You'd been taking them for a year, you'd been tak[ing it?]

117 P: *[No] no, lo que pasa es lo siguiente: en este*
[No] no, what happened is the following: this

118 *año donde yo trabajo se produjo un problema muy grave=*
year a very serious problem cropped up at work=

119 D: *=Ya/*
=Yeah/

120 P: *Y dentro de ese problema me repercutió a mí=*
And this problem affected me=

121 D: *=Ya=*
=Yeah=

122 P: *=Y eso me alteró, digamo–, el esquema: el sistema nervioso entonce– eso nervioso*
=And, let's say, that upset my system, the nervous system, so because of that

123 *do– día– no dormía en la noche entonce– tuve que[::]*
I couldn't sleep for two nights, so I had [to ::]

124 D: *[Volver a tomar]=*
[Take it again]=

125 P: *=Claro yo no había toma–o: como en 20 año– yo no había toma–o: cosa– de ese tipo:=*
=Precisely. I hadn't taken it for some 20 years, I hadn't taken anything like that:=

In line 124 Dr. Ana offers the *predictable utterance completion* phrase *Volver a tomar* ("Take it again") to indicate that she has not only been listening to David's description of the events that led him to resume the medication, but following the account so closely that she is able to finish the sentence for him. This joint production of the speech occurs after an elongated vowel in the last word (*que::*) of the patient's previous utterance. Ferrara has suggested that use of elongated syllables and vowels indicates "the mutual influence of the rhythmic patterns of speakers" (1992: 220; see also Tannen 1989). As with the previous example, the patient's agreement form *Claro* ("Precisely") in line 125 lets the doctor know that joint production of the discourse was both correct and welcome.

6.2.3 Helpful utterance completion

Only four examples were identifed also of the joint production type that is intended to help the speaker construct and complete the speech. In the following exchange Paola is having difficulty coming up with a lexical term to describe the muscular tightness that is a result of her stress.

Example 58 Consultation N° 14 (Doctor: Carlos, Patient: Paola)

62 P: =*Yo, no soy muy tranquila que digamo– entonces en mi trabajo=*
=I, I'm not, what shall we say, a very relaxed person, so in my work=

63 D: =*Ya=*
=Yeah=

64 P: =*De repente me altero y yo sentía como que esta– parte– de acá como que estaban*
=Sometimes I get stressed, and I was feeling as if these parts (of my body)

65 *así como:*
as if they were like

66 D: *¿apretadas?*
tight?

67 P: *Sí, como apretada– …*
Yes, as if (they were) tight …

The doctor detects from the tentative utterance in line 65 *así como:* ("as if they were like") that Paola is struggling to find the right word and supplies the *helpful utterance completion ¿apretadas?* ("tight?") in line 66. This single vocabulary

Table 18. Discourse strategies used in *Assisting patients' stories*

Joint production	Frequency	%
Utterance extension	17	68
Predictable utterance extension	4	16
Helpful utterance completion	4	16
Invited utterance completion	0	0
TOTAL	25	100

item fills the gap in the patient's narrative and allows her to continue without a shift of footing.

Table 18 indicates that *utterance extension* was the preferred strategy for doctor and patient to contribute to each other's talk and to assist in the production of a collaborative discourse. Ferrara's fourth type, *invited utterance completion*, did not occur in this study.

6.3 Creating empathy with the patient

Analysis of the data identifies two discourse strategies associated with the doctor's efforts to create empathy with the patient. The first of these is the use of *agreement discourse markers* to respond positively to the patient's talk. The second is a *reciprocating* of the patient's emotional utterances, in which the doctor as *Fellow Human* aligns with the personal situation of the patient. These strategies are illustrated through the examples given below.

6.3.1 Agreement discourse markers

Doctors made frequent use of *marcadores pragmáticos de apoyos discursivos* (Pons & Samaniego 1998) ("pragmatic markers to assist the discourse") in their conversations with patients. These are exemplified in Spanish by such words as *Claro* ("Of course/You're right"), which Pons and Samaniego classify as an *apoyador de opinión* ("opinion supporter"). *Exacto* ("Precisely") and *Sí* ("Yes") are also identified as opinion supporters in the data, as are utterances consisting of more than one word to indicate that the doctor agrees with what the patient is saying.

In Example 59 we can see the use of an *agreement discourse marker* to give positive feedback to the patient who is recounting her medical history.

Example 59 Consultation Nº 3 (Doctor: Ana, Patient: Carmen)

249 D: *Lo terminó (el medicamento), por eso se lo dejaron los ginecólogos para justamente*
You've finished (the medication), that's why the gynaecologist prescribed it for you,

250 *evitar este problema, pero Uste– me dice que ya no lo siente tan seguido*
to prevent precisely that problem, but you're telling me that you don't feel it (the discomfort) so often now

251 P: *No porque no he ido má–. Tenía que ir este me–*
I don't, and that's why I haven't gone again. I had to go this month,

252 *me iban a dar una– hormona –no sé que diantre=*
they were going to prescribe me some hormones or something like that=

253 D: *=Exacto, justamente se usan hormona– para evitar esto– problema–=*
=Precisely, hormones are used precisely to prevent that problem=

254 P: *=Ya=*
Yeah=

The doctor's *Exacto* ("Precisely") in line 253 supports Carmen's recollection of the gynaecologist's advice and functions to encourage her to feel that she is competent in understanding her hormonal problem. *Exacto* can be interpreted as showing empathy in the form of praise.

Agreement discourse markers may also be employed to show an appreciation of the patient's lifestyle issues rather than simply to confirm medical facts. In the next example Carmen is explaining why she has not made the appointment for a counselling session.

Example 60 Consultation Nº 3 (Doctor: Ana, Patient: Carmen)

110 P: *Eh: yo ni siquiera me averigué tengo en todo caso la hojita que Uste– me dio,*
Eh I didn't even make enquires. In any case, I've got the note you gave me,

111 *pero: lo quiero conversar con mi jefe para, pero:: no he podido conversar porque*
but I want to talk it over with my employer but I haven't been able to talk to him because

112 *pasa en [reunione–]*
he's has been in [meetings]

113 D: *[Claro]*
[Right]

The use of *Claro* ("Of course") in line 113 indicates that the doctor recognizes the difficulty the patient has had in talking to her busy employer about the possibility of leaving work early to attend the psychotherapy group, and shows an affiliation and alignment with the patient's problem.

Agreement discourse markers are interactional strategies whose meaning is context-dependent. Those we have identified so far were used to support the patient's factual contribution or assessment of his/her situation, whereas *claro* in the next example has a more empathic force.

Example 61 Consultation Nº 3 (Doctor: Ana, Patient: Carmen)

124 P: *Sí yo pienso, bueno ahora me he da–o cuenta de que me falta que me siento bastante*
Yes, I think, well, I've realized now that I'm missing something, that I'm feeling very

125 *sola y que me falta– amiga– o dónde tener que salir el día sábado o el día domingo*
lonely and that I don't have a friend or anywhere to go on Saturday or Sunday.

126 *porque por último que no haga toda– la– cosa– en mi casa, pero po– poder salir un*
I don't mind if I don't do all my housework, but at least to be able to go somewhere for

127 *rato digamo–*
a short time

128 D: *Claro, eso, eso en ese senti–o la va a apoyar la psicoterapia ahora ...*
You're right, the psychotherapy group will help you in that regard ...

In line 128 the *agreement discourse marker* is used in the sense of both (a) "I understand how lonely you feel and I sympathize" (empathy marker); and (b) "You're right in your reflection on your needs, and I share your view" (empathy and agreement marker). The *Fellow Human voice* thus acknowledges the patient's emotions and validates the thoughts and feelings she is putting forward. We can contrast this extract with Example 6 in Chapter 4, in which Dr. Ana in the *Doctor voice* was concerned only with Carmen's *physical* symptoms of nausea and diarrhoea.

Empathy can also be shown with an affiliative utterance rather than a single word, as demonstrated in this exchange between Dr. Berta and her patient.

Example 62 Consultation Nº 9 (Doctor: Berta, Patient: Javiera)

48 D: *Ya aquí estaba (la presión) en 110 siempre. Vamos a ver como están las presione– ahora*
O.K., your blood pressure was always at 110. We'll check to see how it is now

49 P: *Venía al sol y eso yo creo que me sube la presión porque se me calienta mucho*
I was walking along in the sun and I think my blood pressure goes up because my

50 *la cabeza porque por Vicuña Mackenna da todo el sol y que <WH quemaba WH>*
head gets very hot, because along Vicuña Mackenna you get the full sun <WH it was burning WH>.

51 *increíble que tan temprano quemando tan fuerte el sol=*
It's unbelievable that the sun was so strong so early on=

52 D: *=Sí, sí y uno ya anda má– o meno– desabrigada bueno se supone que estamos*
=Yes, yes and we wear light dresses. Well, we think we're in

53 *en primavera pero como fue la lluvia pasada digamo– con trueno– con relámpago–=*
spring, but the last time it rained we had thunder and lightning=

The doctor's *Sí, sí* ("Yes, yes") in line 52 indicates that she is listening to Javiera's account and agrees with her about the hot weather. This simple *agreement marker* is then reinforced in lines 52–53 with further remarks on the erratic weather the city has been experiencing during the spring. (Thunder and lightning are unusual conditions for the brightest and most colourful season in Santiago.) By volunteering this extended conversation on the weather, Dr. Berta may be hoping to put her patient at ease before taking her blood pressure. Javiera herself had raised the topic as a concern, believing that it was having a negative impact on her health.

This example reveals that although the doctor's *medical* objective is to perform a routine test (i.e. check the patient's blood pressure), an extended affiliative utterance beforehand to indicate sensitivity to the patient's feelings can be helpful in achieving this objective while putting the patient at ease. (On the use of affiliative strategies to minimize patient discomfort in a particular medical event, see also Aronsson & Rundström 1989; Grainger 2002; Haakana 2001; Roter & Hall 1992.)

6.3.2 Emotional reciprocity

Emotional reciprocity is another strategy to denote affiliation with the patient. This is achieved with discourse features that convey an emotional response to aspects of the patient's story.

Example 63 Consultation Nº 5 (Doctor: Ana, Patient: Esteban)

7 P: *... La verda– que me tardé un poco en venir porque, bueno*
... The truth is that I delayed a little in coming because,

8 *ah: tocó pa' empezar se me: complicó la salu– de mi señora=*
well, to start with, my wife hasn't been well=

9 *=Ah /ya*
=Ah /yeah\

10 P: *Y despué– tuve una tía de 82 año– que le dio como trombosi– =*
And then I had my aunt who is 82 with thrombosis=

11 D: *=[Ah:/ ya\]*
=[Ah:/ yeah\]

12 P: *[Justo ese] día del dieciocho=*
[Exactly] on the 18th=[1]

13 D: *=Claro, sí, pero [la tuvieron ahí]*
=Alright, yes, but [they had her there]

14 P: *[Así que la tuvimo–] que llevar pa' la casa despué–, estuvo*
[So afterwards we had to] take her back home, and she stayed

15 *como quince día– con nosotro– en la casa*
with us for some fifteen days.

16 D: *Ya ... ¡chu:ta!*
Yeah ... Oh gosh!

The colloquial expression *Ya ¡chuta!* ("Yeah Oh gosh!"[2]) in line 16 expresses the doctor's emotional reaction to the difficulties the patient has experienced as a result of the ill-health of his wife and aunt. This spontaneous shift to a register found in everyday conversation, including a colloquial expression such as *¡chuta!*, brings the *Fellow Human voice* to the fore and allows the doctor to show affiliation with the patient by removing the constraints imposed by the strictly medical discourse. Beach (2001: 230) indicates that, in the case of delivering and receiving bad news during the consultation, *relational* issues are

Table 19. Discourse strategies used in *Creating empathy*

Agreement markers	Frequency	%
Exacto	17	30.9
Sí	10	18.2
Claro	19	34.5
Extended agreement	5	9.1
Emotional reciprocity	4	7.3
TOTAL	55	100

usually at stake. For the doctor at these moments, finding the right *voice* can be crucial.

> One "barometer" of intimacy, for example, is a greater likelihood that identification with a situation is revealed through actions tailored to that persons' circumstances (e.g., through sympathy, compassion, excitement, willingness to help through caregiving). (2001:230)

Table 19 shows that empathy was conveyed through single words in 83.6% of cases, while a more involved response occured only 9 times (16.4%).

6.4 Showing special attentiveness to patients' stories

Doctors have recourse to two further discourse strategies to demonstrate their attentiveness and interest and to allow and encourage their patients to take their turn in the discourse. One of these is repetition of the patient's last word(s) (*mirroring*), while the other seeks *clarification* of the patient's previous utterance.

6.4.1 Mirroring

I use the concept of *mirroring* (as a synonym of echoing) in this study following Coates, who describes this speech behaviour as "reciprocal self-disclosure" (1996:61). Coates points out that sometimes utterance mirroring is "so carefully done" (1996:80) that participants will start the utterance with the same phrase and use the same discourse forms. This is precisely what was found in this study. The examples below show mirroring in practice.

Example 64 Consultation Nº 11 (Doctor: Carlos, Patient: Manuel)

32 D: *Mm ya, ya. Vio también el urólogo. Lo encontraron bastante bien.*
Mm yeah, yeah. You saw the urologist as well. They reported that you were quite well.

33 *Oftalmología y a cirugía ¿no ha ido?*
You haven't been to Opthalmology or Surgery?

34 P: *No <@@>*
No <@@>

35 D: *Ya. ¿Le tiene temor?*
Yeah. Are you frightened?

36 P: *No, lo que pasa es que doctor es que no hay tiempo=*
No, what happens, doctor, is that there's no time=

37 D: *=No hay tiempo=*
=There's no time=

38 P: *=Estoy trabajando todavía [y te]ngo*
=I'm still working [and I']ve

39 D: *[Y/a]*
[Y/eah]

40 P: *mucha responsabilida– incluso estoy tan nervio=*
a lot of responsibility, and I'm feeling very tense=

...

133 D: *=¿Y uste– ¿cuándo se da cuenta que está má–, má– las narice– má– tapa–a–?*
=And when do you realize that your nose is more, more, more blocked?

134 P: *Hue– en, en la noche=*
Well at night=

135 D: *=En la noche=*
=At night=

136 P: *=Cuando ya uno ya descansa ya=*
=When one's already resting=

The use of mirroring is first shown in line 37 where the doctor latches onto the patient's phrase *no hay tiempo* ("there isn't time") and uses an exact repetition of the utterance. This has the effect of accelerating the conversation but does not disrupt the patient's account, which continues in line 38. Similarly, in line 135 the doctor repeats the patient's *en la noche* ("at night"), also by latching onto his previous turn. In both cases the mirroring encourages the patient by letting him know that the doctor is following his words closely and expects him to go on describing his symptoms. This strategy is demonstrated again in the following exchange between Dr. Daniel and Yolanda, although this time there is no latching and the patient terminates the episode.

Example 65 Consultation Nº 21 (Doctor: Daniel, Patient: Yolanda)

153 D: *=¿Cuándo vio al doc[tor?]*
=When did you see the doc[tor?]

154 P: *[Cuando] fui a la consulta, ¿sí?*
[When] did I go to consult him, you mean?

155 D: *Sí*
Yes

156 P: *Hace como quince día–*
Some fifteen days ago

157 D: *Quince día–*
Fifteen days

158 P: *Mm*
Mm

159 D: *¿Y hace cuánto– año– o mese– llevaba tomándolo?*
And how many years or months have you been taking it?

Here the doctor mirrors the patient's *quince día–* ("fifteen days") in line 157 but the patient chooses not to take the next turn. Instead she utters only the *agreement marker Mm*. This indicates that she wants the doctor to initiate the next episode, which he then does in line 159 with a *QSI one* in the *Doctor voice*.

In contrast to this, let us look at an example where the doctor uses mirroring to *halt* the patient's words even though it is clear that the patient has not completed his utterance.

Example 66 Consultation Nº 10 (Doctor: Carlos, Patient: Leonel)

41 D: *[¿Y ahí] estaba tomando uno completo?*
[And then] you were taking a whole tablet?

42 P: *Uno completo, sí. Y el fraccionado*
A whole tablet, yes. And half of it

43 D: *Fraccionado y ¿ese malestar cuánto tiempo le duró?*
Half of it, and how long did the discomfort last?

The use of *fraccionado* ("half of it") in line 43 shows that the doctor has been attentive to what the patient has just said, but the purpose of the mirroring is not to facilitate the patient's next turn. Rather it places a stop-sign in the patient's speech and gives the green light to the *Doctor voice* to retake the floor using a *QSI one*. *Mirroring* is therefore a listening strategy that indicates that the doctor is paying particularly close attention to the patient's words. It can function similarly to a *continuer marker* in encouraging the patient to proceed with the narrative, but it can also be used by doctors as a polite way of blocking the patient's next turn and introducing a shift of footing.

6.4.2 Clarifying a previous utterance

During the consultation the doctor may ask a question to clarify something that the patient has said. This form of questioning differs from the *QSI* we encountered earlier in the *Doctor voice*, in which the patient was addressed simply as a source of information: the doctor initiated the episode by seeking specific medical facts that he/she wanted from the patient to help with assessment and treatment. Here in the *Fellow Human voice* the purpose of the question is to ensure that the doctor has understood the information the patient him/herself has volunteered. The difference between these two types of question is made clear in the following example.

Example 67 Consultation N° 12 (Doctor: Carlos, Patient: Nicolás)

95 D: *¿Y la Ranitidina?*
And the Ranitidina?

96 P: *Esa la tomo en la noche eh: porque en la mañana …*
I take it at night time eh: because in the morning …

97 *o sea no sé que será que me hace evacuar en la mañana*
I don't really know (what happens) but during the morning it makes my bowels open

98 D: *¿La Ranitidina?*
Ranitidina?

In line 95 the doctor asks a *QSI* to determine the patient's compliance in taking a particular medication. The patient responds in the affirmative, but goes on to describe how he has modified his medication because of symptoms of discomfort (lines 96–97). The doctor's next question *¿La Ranitidina?* in line 98 is not a further enquiry regarding compliance but a cautionary utterance that they are both referring to the same medication. The question is prompted by the doctor's concern to achieve his professional goal of providing proper medical

Table 20. Discourse strategies used in *Showing special attentiveness*

Form of special attentiveness	Frequency	%
Mirroring	31	64.6
Clarifying	17	35.4
TOTAL	48	100

care, but it also lets Nicolás know that the doctor is working with his story to ensure informed and appropriate treatment.

Table 20 shows that *mirroring* was used in roughly two-thirds and *clarifying* in about one-third of cases in which doctors demonstrated special attentiveness.

6.5 Asking questions unrelated to the patient's health

The study also revealed that doctors ask questions which do not relate exclusively to medical matters, but touch on work, lifestyle, family, friends or social activities. In the following extract the patient has introduced into the conversation the problems her husband is experiencing. Instead of re-directing the discourse back to the patient's own ongoing symptoms and follow-up management (she has headaches, stomachaches and heart problems), Dr. Daniel opens up Yolanda's story by asking more about her husband's health and offers a supportive ear as she recounts the situation at home.

Example 68 Consultation Nº 21 (Doctor: Daniel, Patient: Yolanda)

77 D: *¿Y su marido por qué sufre tantos cambio– de ánimo?, ¿Ante– no tenía eso?*
And why is your husband suffering so many changes of mood? Did he not have them before?

78 P: *No:: es que Pedro tuvo un, un mucho ¿cómo lo llama Uste–? es trom– son no,*
No:: the fact is that Pedro had a very – how do you call it? a throm– , not a

79 *no trombosis esa grande NO, la chica*
thrombosis the big one NO, a small one

80 D: *Ya, [sí]*
Yeah, [yes]

81 P: *[Vario] a raíz de eso estuvo hospitaliza–o en el, en la Católica*
[A number of them]. For that reason, he was admitted to the Catholic Hospital

82 *hace tres año– ((Carraspera)), va a venir a verlo ah porque él mismo quería,*
three years ago. ((Clearing her throat)) He'll be coming to see you because he himself

83 *que quería ver médico, entonces le había pedido así al lote no má–*
told me that he wanted to make an appointment with a doctor. He asked me for an appointment with anyone (here in the centre)

84 *le dije no porqué no pides hora con el doctor Ponce*[3] *[le dije y así]*
I said to him why don't you make an appointment with doctor Ponce [I told him and so]

85 D: *[¿Y el también] de esto fuera de estos cambio*
[And he also] Apart from these mood

86 *de ánimo eh tiene buena expresión está bien orienta–o no se pierde ni na–a?*
changes, eh does he look alright, is he well oriented, does he get lost or anything like that?

87 P: *No no no eso no=*
No no no, not that=

88 D: *=Ya*
=Yeah=

Dr. Daniel invites Yolanda to talk more about her husband by asking specific questions in lines 77 and 86. Although in each case these take the form of a *QSI chain*, their function can be interpreted not as wanting to seek detailed answers to each question in the chain, but indicating to Yolanda the extent of his empathy and involvement. During her two extended episodes of reply to these questions, he utters only the continuer marker *Ya* ("Yeah") in lines 80 and 88 to let her know that he is listening and to encourage her to go on.

In addition to developing an empathic relationship with his patient through use of these discourse strategies of the *Fellow Human voice*, Dr. Daniel will also have gained a better understanding of the context in which Yolanda's specific health problems are manifested. This awareness could contribute to making a more informed prognosis and formulating a better treatment regimen by taking into account the conditions of her daily life. It is well documented that social factors have a direct bearing on a person's health (Navarro 1990; Pollard 1999; Roter et al. 1992; Sundquist 1995; Waitzkin 1985). Thus, although questions about Yolanda's husband may appear at first sight to be pe-

Table 21. The types of questions doctors ask

Type of question	Frequency	%
QSI in *Doctor voice*	356	93.93
QSI in *Fellow Human voice*	23	6.07
TOTAL	379	100

ripheral to the medical discourse, they may in fact lead to greater effectiveness in managing her health condition.

Table 21 shows the relative frequencies of questions directly related to medical aspects of the patient's self (in the *Doctor voice*, cf. Table 8) and questions relating to broader issues of the patient's lifeworld (*Fellow Human voice*). As one would expect from health practitioners working within the bio-medical frame, the vast majority of doctors' questions focus directly on the information that is required to make a correct diagnosis of the patient's condition and confirm the efficacy of the prescribed treatment and management.

6.6 Statistical findings

As we have seen, doctors make use of various discourse strategies associated with the functions of the *Fellow Human voice* during the history-taking and management routines of the consultation. These include *continuer markers*, *joint production* forms (following Ferrara 1992), *agreement markers*, *mirroring*, *clarifying questions*, *empathic utterances*, and questions designed to understand the patient's health problem in a more holistic framework. In all, a total of 21 out of the 22 consultations in this study were found to contain examples of the *Fellow Human voice*.

The functions *Creating empathy with the patient* and *Showing special attentiveness to patients' stories* were noted in 16 consultations, though not always together in the same consultation. The functions least represented were *Asking questions unrelated to patients' health* (N = 33) and *Assisting the telling of patients' stories* (N = 25). Only 8 consultations included this latter function, and a closer look at the data reveals that the majority of these involved Dr. Carlos, who was responsible for 68% (17/25) of the joint production forms.

Table 22 identifies usage patterns of each of these five functions among the four doctors. Dr. Ana (Total N = 147) and Dr. Carlos (Total N = 182) engaged the *Fellow Human voice* far more frequently than their other two colleagues, Dr. Berta and Dr. Daniel, who recorded totals of 26 and 57 respectively. These

Table 22. Functions of the *Fellow Human voice*: frequencies for individual doctors

Doctor	n	Facilitating the telling of patients' stories		Assisting the telling of patients' stories		Creating empathy with the patient		Showing special attentiveness to patients' stories		Asking questions unrelated to the patients' health		Total
		N	M	N	M	N	M	N	M	N	M	
Dr Ana	6	94	15.6	4	0.6	31	5.1	14	2.3	4	0.6	147
Dr. Berta	3	13	4.3	0	0	5	1.6	4	1.3	4	1.3	26
Dr. Carlos	6	113	18.8	17	2.8	13	2.1	27	4.5	12	2.0	182
Dr. Daniel	7	41	5.8	4	0.5	6	0.8	3	0.4	3	0.4	57
TOTAL		261	63.4%	25	6.0%	55	13.3%	48	11.7%	23	5.6%	412

n = number of consultations
N = frequency
M = mean frequency per consultation

relativities are not altered after taking into account the number of consultations (n). *Facilitating the telling of patients' stories* was the function most used by the four doctors, with a relative frequency of 63.4%. The second most widely used function was *Creating empathy with the patient*, with a relative frequency of 13.3%. The other three functions, which call for more verbal effort on the part of the doctor, had lower frequencies of 6.0%, 11.7% and 5.6%.

Table 23 summarizes the data distribution according to gender. The interesting pattern can be observed that male doctors use the *Fellow Human voice* more frequently when addressing their female patients (Dr. Carlos 99/83 and Dr. Daniel 41/16). A closer scrutiny indicates that the function *Facilitating the telling of patients' stories* is largely responsible for this pattern, with a 64/49 ratio for Dr. Carlos and 31/10 for Dr. Daniel.

Although this pattern is quite distinctive, it does not tell us much about the reasons for this behaviour. In looking for a possible causal link, I then revisited each individual male doctor/female patient dyad and found that almost half of Dr. Carlos's total score of 64 could be accounted for in the one consultation, and similarly with Dr. Daniel, who used this function 17 times with the one female patient out of his overall total of 31. I then wondered whether there could be any common characteristics between these two patients to explain the doctors' high use of *continuer markers* and *receipt markers* in listening to their stories. Both of these female patients were engaged in home duties, without a paid job outside the home, one aged between 41 and 50 and the other over 71 years; however, other women at home did not elicit the same response from the doctors, and age was also discounted. It appeared that my results were bound to the nature of the discourse itself, and not necessarily to sociological factors such as age or occupation. The explanation had to be sought, therefore, at the interactional level of the encounter. These two female patients were dynamic participants in the discourse: they initiated the talk and questioned their doctors on a number of issues. (Both these women, in fact, made the highest use of the *Initiator voice*, to be discussed in the next chapter.) Thus, the *Fellow Human voice* was most likely to function to further the patient's story when the consultation already took the form of a mutually participatory exchange.

Table 23 otherwise shows a fairly evenly matched distribution of functions based on patient gender. Both Dr. Ana and Dr. Berta used discourse strategies to *create empathy* with their patients as the second-highest function of their *Fellow Human voice*, and Dr. Ana was particularly supportive when her male patients expressed emotional difficulties (19 occurrences), as we saw in the passage with Estaban in Example 63 above. Whether the trends found in this

Table 23. Functions of the *Fellow Human voice*: frequencies for individual doctors and male/female patients

Function	Dr. Ana		Dr. Berta	Dr. Carlos		Dr. Daniel		Total
	F (n=3)	M (n=3)	F (n=3)	F (n=3)	M (n=3)	F (n=4)	M (n=3)	
Facilitating the telling of patients' stories								
N	46	48	13	64	49	31	10	261
M	15.3	16.0	4.3	21.3	16.3	7.7	3.3	63.4%
Assisting the telling of patients' stories								
N	3	1	0	7	10	1	3	25
M	1.0	0.3	0.0	2.3	3.3	0.2	1.0	6.0%
Creating empathy with the patient								
N	12	19	5	6	7	4	2	55
M	4.0	6.3	1.6	2.0	2.3	1.0	0.6	13.3%
Showing special attentiveness to patients' stories								
N	7	7	4	16	11	3	0	48
M	2.3	2.3	1.3	5.3	3.6	0.7	0.0	11.7%
Asking questions unrelated to the patients' health								
N	2	2	4	6	6	2	1	23
M	0.6	0.6	1.3	2.0	2.0	0.5	0.3	5.6%
TOTAL	70	77	26	99	83	41	16	412 (100%)

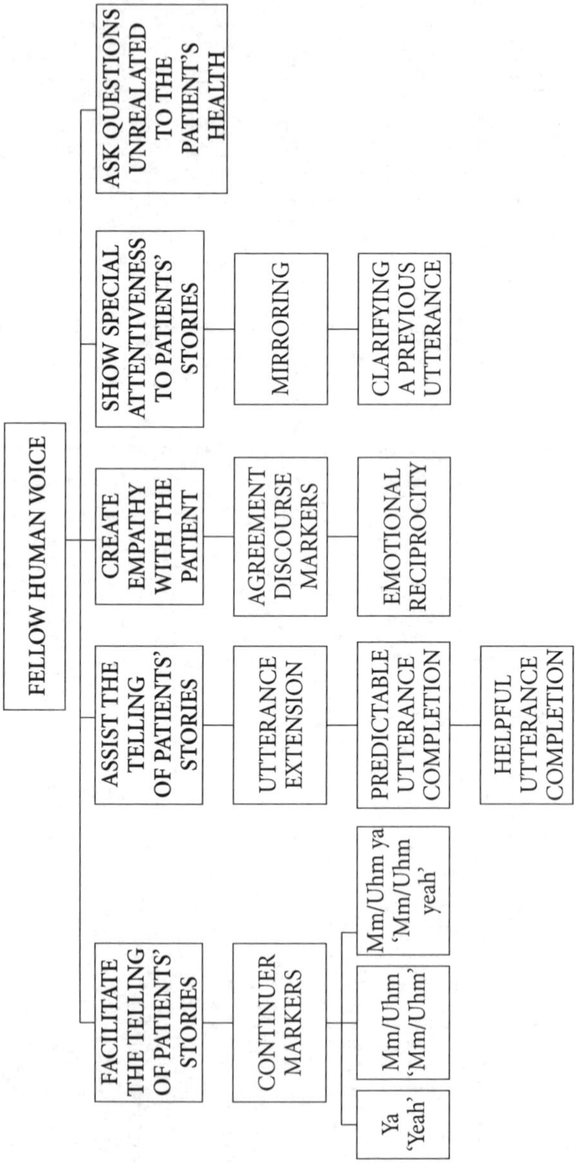

Figure 5. Discourse functions and strategies of *Fellow Human voice*

analysis are of sociological relevance, however, is a question that must await further investigation with a larger sample size.

6.7 Conclusion

Using the five functions of the *Fellow Human voice* explored in this chapter, doctors and patients develop personal connections through discourse. The strategies of this voice are numerous and diverse, but all have the similar aim of showing empathy. The presence of the *Fellow Human* is fundamental to a consultation that views the patient as a *person* as well as a *medical problem* to be treated. And, as we have seen, lifestyle issues revealed in asking questions not of a strictly medical nature can often shed light on the broader cause of the physical complaint and problems with compliance (Frankel 1984, 1990). Further, by feeling that they are listened to, understood and cared for – not just as unwell persons but as individuals who matter (but just happen to be sick) – patients may feel that the consultation is a safe place to share their personal and sometimes difficult stories, which in turn may enhance the medical outcome. Perhaps not surprisingly, the *Fellow Human voice* was identified in all but one of the 22 consultations in this study, indicating that it plays an integral role in doctor–patient relationships.

Figure 5 illustrates the discourse functions and strategies of the *Fellow Human voice*.

Over the previous three chapters we have deconstructed the medical discourse to identify three distinctive *voices* that doctors use. Each *voice* has particular functions, and these are accomplished through specific discourse strategies. While the *Doctor* and *Educator voices* reinforce the hierarchy of the consultative setting, which places the patient in a more passive role, the *Fellow Human voice* encourages the patient to take the floor, and functions best when the patient initiates the talk. Empathic discourse markers place participants on a more equal footing; though, as we have seen, functions in which the shift is greatest and which require the doctor's most active involvement occur less frequently than simple utterances acknowledging the patient's talk.

We have also identified the fluid nature of doctors' *voices*, and the frequent shifts of footing they exercise in the discourse. These shifts are responses in one way or another to the utterances of the other participant in the exchange – the patient. Accordingly, patients' *voices* and their dynamic relationship with the *Doctor*, *Educator* and *Fellow Human voices* are the subject of the next chapter.

Notes

1. Chileans celebrate Independence Day on the 18th of September.
2. *¡chuta!* does not have the religious derivation of the English translation.
3. The name of the doctor has been changed.

Chapter 7

Patients' *voices*

7.1 Introduction

Having discussed in previous chapters how *doctors* participate in the medical exchange, and how their *voices* align to the medical institution and the socio-cultural group they represent, this chapter puts the "spotlight on the patient" (Drew 2001). What is it that *patients* do in their medical talk? What *voices* do they have? How is their social image of themselves portrayed in their discourse? And how do their *voices* interact with those of their treating physician? In this chapter I shift the focus away from doctors' talk, which has dominated studies of medical discourse, and concentrate instead on the contribution made by the patient. In so doing, I introduce the broader aim of this study, which is to identify *all* the *voices* found in the consultative setting and to understand medical discourse as an essentially *dynamic* process between doctor and patient. While some studies have focused on para-linguistic aspects of patients' talk, and others have noted certain linguistic features in patients' recounting of their stories (Ainsworth-Vaughn 1998; Davis 1988; Labov & Fanshel 1977), the predominance of doctor-based studies has tended to silence patients' voices in the literature (Mishler 1984). In the clinical setting, however, patients' voices may not be so easily suppressed.

Like doctors, patients use different *voices* during the consultation. Although one cannot "learn" to be a patient and there are no guidelines for the role, this study has nonetheless observed some commonalities in the ways patients portray themselves and the kinds of stories they bring to the visit. These patterns exist even when the amount of contact the patient has had with medical treatment differs widely from person to person.

The following patient *voices* have been identified for analysis:

a. The *voice* of *Health-related storytelling*
b. The *voice* of *Competence*
c. The *voice* of *Social Communicator*
d. The *voice* of *Initiator*

With one exception, every consultation I recorded included examples of at least two of the above *voices* in the communication routines of history-taking and management and treatment. (One patient confined himself to recounting his medical history only.) This suggests that patients on the whole did not feel constrained by the clinical setting to conform to a strictly medical discourse. Rather, they felt sufficiently at ease to explore topics of an everyday nature and to present themselves as social beings with individual personalities (*voice* of *Social Communicator*). They also initiated questions to find out more information about their health problem and treatment, and to demonstrate their ability in managing their condition (*voices* of *Initiator* and *Competence*).

Before describing and analysing these four *voices*, it is important to emphasize the interactional nature of storytelling. In the previous chapter we saw that doctors may attach their own motives to the patient's act of sharing their story, such as a desire to create rapport with the patient (Norrick 1997); we have also seen that doctors control the interview and will sometimes check the patient's narrative flow. For their part, patients have to feel a need to share a part of their lives with their doctors; that is, there must be something worthwhile telling (Labov & Fanshel 1977), something unusual that calls for an evaluative point to be made (Davis 1988), a desire for conversation. In addition, as some of the data shows, the patient may wish to project a particular image and does so by *authoring* a preferred script. On the other hand, if the patient shows no interest in developing the story, despite the opportunities to do so, the conversation will not occur. This is the case in the following extract, where the doctor encourages his patient to talk about the difficulty she is having in keeping to her prescribed low-calorie diet – to no avail.

Example 69 Consultation N° 19 (Doctor: Daniel, Patient: Wilma)

17 D: *¿Cómo le ha ido con el peso?*
How's your weight loss been going?

18 P: <@@> *no me ha ido=*
<@@> it's not going=

19 D: *=¿Bajó de peso?*
=Have you lost weight?

20 P: *Sí, parece*
Yes, I think so

21 D: *Sí, bajó <X 66 X>=*
Yes, you've lost <X 66 X>=

22 P: *=Do– no má–=*
=Only two (kilos)=

23 D: *=Poquito pero bajó. Cuénteme y y y eh ¿está tratando de hacer régimen?*
It's a little, but you've lost (some weight). Tell me, and and and you're trying to keep on the diet?

24 *¿Cómo lo ha hecho? eh ¿Qué tanto le ha costado?*
How have you been doing it? How difficult has it been?

25 P: *Eh eh uhm*
Eh eh uhm

26 D: *Ya*
O.K.

27 P: *Na– má– po'*
That's all

28 D: *¿Anda con ansieda– de comer?*
Do you have any yearning to eat?

Dr. Daniel initiates this conversation with a *QSI one* in line 17, asking his patient for a report on her progress with the low-calorie diet. The incomplete reply in line 18, which simply mirrors the doctor's question as a negative by including *no*, together with a laugh at the beginning of the utterance, suggests that Wilma feels uncomfortable with the subject. Clearly, the diet "is not going" (anywhere). Dr. Daniel then tries again, using a second *QSI one* in line 19. The patient answers *Sí, parece* ("Yes, I think so") in line 20, but this minimal response again indicates a reluctance to elaborate on the subject. The doctor then shifts to making an assessment of her progress *Sí, bajó ...* ("Yes, you've lost ...") in line 21 – after all, she has lost *some* weight – but the patient cuts off his attempt at positive feedback with the negating *Do– no má–* ("Only two (kilos)") in line 22. A new discourse strategy is tried in lines 23–24 with a *QSI chain*, the real purpose of which, as we saw in Example 68 in the previous chapter, is not to seek factual information, but to convey the doctor's concern for the patient and willingness to try different strategies to elicit her contribution. The empathy of the question *¿qué tanto le ha costado?* ("How difficult has it been?") reinforces this intention. Wilma's non-committal reply in line 25, however, and then her utterance in line 27 *Na– má– po'* ("That's all") with the discourse marker *po'*, show a decisiveness (Pons & Samaniego 1998) about her non-cooperation. This leaves the doctor no choice but to begin the cycle again with a *QSI one* in line 28.

Wilma's case exemplifies the collaborative effort that is required for the production of the patient's story, as well as the power that both participants have to either enable or constrain the storytelling. From the doctor's perspective, on the one hand there is a medical imperative to listen to the patient's history, while on the other there are constraints both in the medical system and in the context of the consultation that affect the number of turns the patients can be allocated. From the patient's point of view, the *voice* of *Health-related storytelling* must be asserted if the presenting health problem or symptoms are to be alleviated; however, this *voice* may be suppressed if the patient feels uncomfortable with or embarrassed by the information that is sought, or if the doctor fails to establish sufficient rapport with the patient or sends out signals that cast doubt on the validity of the patient's contribution.

The following example shows how the doctor validates the patient's story by showing genuine respect and understanding as she makes her own evaluation of the effect spring has had on her health.

Example 70 Consultation Nº 21 (Doctor: Daniel, Patient: Yolanda)

24 D: *¿Su ánimo?* How are you feeling?

25 P: *Eh: mi ánimo ya está subiendo un poco, sí, es que sabe, doctor, a mí me afecta*
Eh: my spirits are getting a little better; yes, you know, doctor, all that affects me

26 *todo ésto, me afecta mucho la::=*
it affects me a lot=

27 D: *=Ya=*
=Yeah=

28 P: *=Siempre me afectó la primavera y este año como tuvimo– primavera invierno,*
=Spring has always affected me, and this year, because we had spring winter

29 *primavera invierno, como que se me pegó un poco. NO, pero ahora sí estoy ya*
spring winter, my problem persisted a little. NO, but now I'm coming out of it, I'm not

30 *saliendo, ya no estoy haciendo sie:sta*
having my (usual) nap

31 D: *Pero le afecta la primavera. ¿Cuándo llega la primavera le baja el ánimo?*
But spring affects you. When spring arrives, you feel down?

32 P: *Sí <@@> ¡qué tontera! ¿no? <@@>*
Yes <@@> how silly of me! Don't you think? <@@>

33 D: *No [no tiene na–a de tontera]*
No [no, it's not silly at all]

34 P: *[Me parece que] no e– normal eh: no sé, y desde joven ah, se me había– pasa–o*
[It seems to me that] it's not normal eh. I don't know, and I've been like that since I was young

35 D: *Ya*
Yeah

36 P: *Pero::*
But::

37 D: *¿Y cómo ha esta–o de la– jaqueca–?*
How have the migraines been?

In line 33 the utterance *No no tiene na–a de tontera* ("No, no, it's not silly at all") not only reassures Yolanda that her self-evaluation is being taken seriously, but also establishes a platform of affiliative understanding for expanding the boundaries of the speech. Yolanda feels comfortable and continues her commentary in line 34. Had Dr. Daniel laughed in line 32 along with his patient (Davis 1988), or offered only a simple *continuer marker*, Yolanda may have interpreted this as agreeing that her account was foolish and of little value. This would most likely have had a negative and constraining effect on the discourse.

7.2 The *voice* of *Health-related storytelling*

The patient's *voice* of *Health-related storytelling* has a functional relationship with the *Doctor voice*, which seeks information about the patient's health. 61 examples of this patient *voice* were identified in 17 of the consultations of this study. Patients develop their *Health-related storytelling* by:

a. Describing their emotional state (e.g. *me siento depre*, "I feel depressed"; *me siento bajoneá*, "I feel down").
b. Describing their physical symptoms, such as discomfort or pain (e.g. *dolor de estómago*, "stomach ache"; *dolor de cabeza*, "headache").
c. Expressing concern about their health condition, treatment or management (e.g. *temor a la operación*, "worry about having the operation").
d. Sharing their difficulties in complying with medical recommendations (e.g. *dejar de fumar*, "quit smoking").

Health-related storytelling is usually triggered by a doctor's *QSI*, which may be of a general nature (e.g. *¿Su ánimo?*, "How are you feeling?") or addressed to a specific aspect of the patient's history (e.g. *¿Cuándo se hizo Uste– el examen?*, "When did you have your last test?"). *Continuer markers* and other affirmative utterances by both doctors and patients enable the narrative to be elaborated and extended.

As noted above, *Health-related storytelling* is generally employed in combination with one or more of the other three patient *voices* in the discourse. The main characteristic of this *voice* is that it articulates a past experience and does so in more than one utterance. In terms of its temporal structure, *Health-related storytelling* is identified by use of the past tense for the event(s) being described and by a comparison of the patient's past and present states of being. Adverbs of time such as *antes* ("before") and *ahora* ("now") are common in the discourse. Markers of inclusion such as *mire* ("look"), *imagínese* ("imagine yourself") and *¿sabe?* ("you know?") at the beginning or in the middle of utterances serve as brief pauses in the speech to confirm the hearer's attention, to emphasize that the story is worth the telling, and to indicate that it will be further developed. "A central fact about all of these affective propositions is that they revolve about the social concept of 'reportability'" (Labov & Fanshel 1977: 105).

Health-related storytellers present themselves, perforce, as people who seek assistance for a personal problem they lack the expertise to manage on their own. As Davis (1988: 253) has suggested, "the issue of needing help is a potentially problematic affair". Attached to an admission of inability to care for and manage oneself may be the fear of projecting a lack of adult competence (Labov & Fanshel 1977: 32) and "losing face" (Brown & Levinson 1987; Goffman 1967). This imbalance in the doctor–patient relationship is precisely what sets the medical consultation apart from other forms of interaction and explains why patients may call on other *voices* to compensate for the asymmetry of their *Health-related storyteller* status in the exchange. In addition, the other *voices* may be a response to the doctor's individual consulting style, whether one that favours a strict medical agenda (*Doctor voice*) or one that is sensitive to the patient's more vulnerable role and engages in discourse related to their lifeworld (Mishler 1984).

In the following example the patient talks about his constant fear when carrying out even the most ordinary of daily activities, such as going into the backyard or taking out the rubbish.

Example 71 Consultation Nº 12 (Doctor: Carlos, Patient: Nicolás)

169 P: *... me empiezo a agitar ya cuando voy al fondo del patio*
... I begin to get agitated even when I go to the back of my yard

a hacer alguna cosa sacar la basura
to do anything to take the rubbish out

170 D: *Ya*
Yeah

...

179 P: *Es que yo tuve un problema ha: mucho– año–. Yo le temo, no me subo a un:*
The fact is I've had a problem for many years now. I'm scared. I don't take

180 *o sea ascensor, no lo soporto*
a lift, I can't bear it

181 D: *¿Por qué? ¿Por qué es muy est[recho?]*
Why? Is it because it's very na[rrow]

182 P: *[Claro]*
[Precisely]

183 D: *¿O no le gusta como apretado con otra– persona–?*
Or you don't like being hemmed in with other people?

184 P: *Claro,no, no, no. Me da miedo=*
Precisely, no, no, no. I'm afraid=

185 D: *=Uhm ya y Cuándo [va a un lugar]*
=Uhm yeah and when [you go somewhere]

186 P: *[Ahora a Antofagasta] eh: me ofrecieron un viaje que*
[Now I'm going to Antofagasta] eh: I was offered

187 *fuera en avión, pero le tengo terror=*
a plane ticket, but I'm petrified=

188 D: *=Uhm ya=*
=Mm yeah=

189 P: *=Yo no sé porqué son esta– cosa–, pero de [repente]*
=I don't know why this happens, but [suddenly]

190 D: *[¿Ha tenido] alguna experiencia*
[Have you ever had] an unpleasant experience

191 *desagradable en ascensor o en espacio reducido?*
in a lift or in a confined space?

192 P: *Eh: he tenido en ascensor tuve y también en el 73 que no– encerraron en la*
Eh: I've had one in a lift, and also in 73 when we were locked inside

193 *empresa*
the company

194 D: *Ya*
Yeah

195 P: *Y de ahí noté que despué– de ya me vinieron=*
And since then I've noticed this feeling of=

196 D: *=El encierro*
=being enclosed

197 P: *Encierrro y la presión del momento que se estaba vivie:ndo.*
Enclosure and the pressure that people were experiencing at the time

198 *Eso me chocó mucho*
That shocked me greatly

199 D: *Cuénteme, y la ¿sensación de angustia [sen]sación?*
Tell me, are you still feeling anxious [fee]ling?

200 P: *[Sí]*
[Yes]

The patient expresses his feelings in line 169 (*me empiezo a agitar*, "I begin to get agitated"), but he is unable to account for them. His next utterance in line 179 is introduced with the discourse marker *Es que* ("The fact is"), which raises the expectation that he may be going to offer some explanation for the cause of his problems; however, this turns out not to be the case. Getting to the root of the problem requires intensive interactional work on the part of the doctor. He has the double task of "evaluating the trouble as terrible and establishing the trouble teller's need of help" (Davis 1988: 253). In his account, Nicolás describes his feelings of fear in confined spaces, specifically in lifts and planes, but seems powerless to explore the reasons for this (*Yo no sé porqué son esta– cosa–*, "I don't know why this happens") in line 189. His choice of words to describe his emotional distress intensifies the experience: *le temo* ("I'm scared"), *me da miedo* ("I'm afraid"), and even *le tengo terror* ("I'm petrified"). In his *voice* of *Health-related storytelling*, the patient has provided little factual information, but raised a cry for help.

In lines 190–191 Dr. Carlos initiates a *QSI multiple choice* that alludes to Nicolas's earlier admission about his fear of lifts (line 180). This question appears to display affiliation (Jefferson 1984) towards the trouble-talk the patient is referring to, and reassures him that it is "safe" to open up further about his attacks of claustrophia. It proves to be an effective strategy, as the patient then tells the doctor about his traumatic experience in 1973, when he and his colleagues were locked inside the building they were working in during the military coup.[1] The *continuer marker Ya* ("Yeah") in line 194 and the *helpful utterance completion El encierro* ("being enclosed") in line 196 encourage Nicolás to recall the events that led to his panic attacks and to share them with the doctor.

Interestingly, however, in line 199 Dr. Carlos returns the discourse to the present tense with a *QSI one* in the *Doctor voice*, which serves to terminate Nicolás's recollections. It may be that the doctor felt it would not be helpful for his patient to dwell on disturbing past events any longer. Clearly, he is still suffering the long-term effects of his confinement in 1973. Perhaps also, however, the absence of an affiliative discourse on this occasion owes itself to divergent political allegiances. Dr. Carlos may not have wished to be drawn into a conversation on political issues on which he and his patient held different views.

7.3 The *voice* of *Competence*

Patients have been called competent, knowledgeable and "probing" (Fisher 1991; Royster 1990) when they show they are familiar with medical procedures and understand their health condition. For Barton (2000), competent patients are those who follow medical recommendations and accord with medical advice. In this section I will focus on the *voice* of *Competence* by describing and analysing how the patients in this study projected themselves during the consultation.

It became clear that patients could be divided into three distinct groups. The first group were *Compliers*: they understood the doctor's instructions and their own responsibilities and were able to report that they had successfully carried out the required tasks. The second group presented as *Apologizers*: these patients too understood the doctor's instructions, but somewhere along the line their good intentions to carry them out had broken down. The third group were the *Challengers*: these individuals had developed some expertise of their own in the course of becoming competent and responsible for their health, and contested the doctor's recommendations and authority from their new power base of knowledge.

7.3.1 The *Complier*

Compliers are individuals who follow the recommendations given to them and so demonstrate alignment to medical authority. It can be assumed that doctor and patient reached agreement on these recommendations during the previous consultation. Bissell et al. (2003) refer to this mutual negotation during the medical interview as "concordance".

In the following example Javiera presents herself as a model of compliance in her follow-up visit to Dr. Berta.

Example 72 Consultation Nº 9 (Doctor: Berta, Patient: Javiera)

26 P: =*(Tomo la medicina) media hora antes de la comi–a tal como Uste– me dijo*
=(I take the medicine) half an hour before eating, as you told me to

27 D: *Ya perfecto y ¿qué toma para la <X X> de azúcar?*
Right, perfect. And what are you taking as a sub <X X> for sugar?

28 P: *Eh Nutrasuit*
Eh Nutrasuit

29 D: *Ah ya*
Ah yeah

30 P: *Y hago el régimen TAL CUAL me lo indicaron en el hospital*
And I'm following the diet PRECISELY as it was given to me in the hospital

31 D: *Uhm ya*
Uhm yeah

32 P: *En ese sentido no quiero que nada me tiente. Ya no voy a dejar . . .*
In that regard I don't want anything tempting. I won't give up . . .

In the first line of this extract the patient tells her doctor that she has been taking the medication *tal como Uste– me dijo* ("as you told me to"). This utterance makes explicit her acknowledgement of the doctor's role of authorizing treatment and the patient's role of complying with that treatment. The patient also shows a similar alignment to the hospital where she had been admitted in the past (line 30). This time the emphatic adverbial phrase *TAL CUAL* ("PRECISELY") is included in the utterance, and spoken in a loud voice, to further intensify her account of co-operation (Davis 1988). This image of perfect compliance is reinforced again in the last line, concluding with the dramatic *Ya no voy a dejar . . .* ("I won't give up . . .") in line 32.

The main characteristic of the *Complier* to emerge from this example is a sense of being in control. *Compliers* inform themselves of the requirements for looking after their health, and can demonstrate personal satisfaction and a sense of achievement when they "have it in their power" to contribute to their well-being. Further, by being compliant, doctor and patient enjoy a mutual alignment to the medical establishment, reducing the risk of conflict and instability in their allocated roles.

Patient competence can also enhance doctor–patient communication and contribute to a more successful outcome. Competent patients not only show alignment to the medical institution and its principles of care, but establish a platform for further education to be developed in the discourse. This is so, since the time the doctor might have spent educating the patient about basic requirements can be used to deal with the same or other health issues in greater depth. As a result of this positive and reciprocal feedback, greater success may be expected with the treatment overall.

Example 73 Consultation N° 18 (Doctor: Daniel, Patient: Victor)

63 D: ... *Tolera bien el regimen, no anda con mucha hambre eh: ¿Cómo ha sido éso?*
... Do you put up with the diet easily? Aren't you very hungry? How has it been?

64 P: *Doctor, le digo de que sí ando con hambre y he bajado bastante, por lo que*
Doctor I can tell you that I certainly feel hungry, but I've lost (weight),

65 *Uste– puede ver al al control de hoy día=*
as you can see today=

66 D: =*Uhm=*
=Mm=

67 P: =*Estoy en 64 kilo–, y anteriormente, el otro control lo debe tener por ahí.*
=I'm 64 kilos, and at the previous check-up, you should have it somewhere

68 *Creo que eran cincuenta y, o sea, sesenta y:=*
I think it was fifty, it means sixty=

69 D: =*Setenta tiene aquí=*
=Seventy is (written) here=

70 P: =*Setenta cuando me empezó a tratar. Claro sí, he bajado.*
=Seventy in my first check-up with you, I've clearly lost (weight)

71 *Y me he mantenido, no he subi–o*
I've watched myself myself, and I haven't put on any

72 D: *¿Solamente con dieta?*
Just by following a diet?

73 P: *Solamente con dieta -toy*
I'm just following a diet

74 D: *Yo lo encuentro bastante bien po' ¿Ah? Con la glicemia que trae lleva en forma*
I think it is very good Ah? The result of the glycemia test shows that you're

75 *muy correcta el regimen. Eh: ... sí, me interesaría saber cómo, cómo sigue el regimen durante el*
following your diet perfectly. Eh ... yes, I would like to know how, how you follow your diet over

76 *mes, hay un examen que no es ese pa' chequearlo día a día, solamente*
a month, there's a test that isn't the one to check the level every day since

77 *da una fotografía de ese momento solamente, pero hay otro– que, que*
that one gives only a picture at a particular moment, but there's another

78 *evalúa má– o meno– como ha estado dentro del me–*
that checks roughly how you go over a month

We are already familiar with this conversation, which was used to demonstrate both the *Doctor voice* (Example 18) and the *Educator voice* (Example 30). Competence is revealed in the patient's compliance with the diet and an understanding of his weight loss. The doctor's positive assessment is made clear by his use of reassuring utterances such as *lo encuentro bastante bien* ("I think it is very good") and *lleva en forma muy correcta el regimen* ("you're following your diet perfectly"). Because the patient has shown good results and a capacity for learning, the *Educator voice* in lines 76–78 is able to expound a different kind of test available to check glycaemia levels in the blood. The relationship between *Complier* and *Educator* is discussed further in Chapter 9.

7.3.2 The *Apologizer*

Apologizers are *Compliers* who have failed to act: that is, they understood what was required and agreed to do it, but somehow or other have just not followed through. In this situation the patient's *face* (Brown & Levinson 1987, Cordella in press) is under threat, since a lack of compliance may be equated with a lack of ability to meet one's adult responsibilities (Labov & Fanshel 1977). In order to compensate for this, some "remedial work" is necessary, some strategy that allows the patient to "save face". "Remedial work" has the function of changing "the meaning that otherwise might be given to an act, transforming what could be seen as offensive into what can be seen as acceptable" (Goffman 1971: 109). In this study the potentially offensive act is the lack of compliance on the part of the patient. However, it may be preferable for the patient to temporarily "lose face" through the "remedial work" of owning up to the non-compliance rather than threaten the trust of the doctor that is fundamentally important to the success of their ongoing relationship (see Atkinson 1995). The following example illustrates this point.

Example 74 Consultation N° 20 (Doctor: Daniel, Patient: Ximena)

23 P: *Ya, ... me dio un remedio que tenía que haberlo toma–o, haberlo toma–o*
O.K.... You prescribed a medication that I should have taken. I should have taken

24 *la caja que Uste– me dio y despué– compré otra en el sup– no, no tomé*
the packet you gave me, and then I bought another one in the sup– No, I didn't take it

25 *como debería haberlo hecho. Le voy a ser bien honesta ...*
as I should have done. I'll be very honest with you ...

26 *fui a mi médico al que me ve en Osorno*
I went to the doctor who sees me in Osorno

27 *que que cuando yo tengo algo yo lo voy a ver a él*
I go to him when I've got something wrong with me

27 D: *Ya*
Yeah

28 P: *Y él despué– él me dio una receta para que lo compre y la compré*
And, afterwards he gave me a prescription to buy, and I bought it

29 D: *¿La misma?*
The same one?

30 P: *La misma la misma [la misma]*
The same, the same [the same]

31 D: *[Ya]*
[Yeah]

Ximena starts by indicating that she has failed to comply with the doctor's instructions (presumably given at her last visit). This is expressed in lines 23–24 as an "indirect apology": she acknowledges that she understood the instructions and blames only herself for not following them, but omits from her speech the verb that enacts the apology. Cordella (1990, 1991, 1992) has categorized Chilean apologies into those that are "direct" and those that are "indirect" following Trosborg (1987). In the first group the verb is explicitly stated in the utterance, e.g. *lo siento* ("I'm sorry"), *discúlpeme* ("I apologize"), whereas in the second group the verb that expresses the apology is not present but explanations, acknowledgements of responsibility and promises of forbearance are used instead.

In the example above Ximena's indirect apology is nonetheless designed to ensure that the doctor–patient relationship is not jeopardized by her non-compliance. Her utterances *como debería haberlo hecho* ("as I should have done") and *Le voy a ser bien honesta* ("I'll be very honest with you") in line 25 affirm her alignment to the medical institution. Her willingness to lose *face* by being fully honest with her doctor is further evidence of the importance she places on the interaction. All ends well in any case, as she tells the doctor that she is now taking the medication on prescription from another doctor (line 28).

7.3.3 The *Challenger*

When conflict occurs, it may be triggered by competent patients whose knowledge of their condition causes them to question the doctor's authority, particularly when the prescribed treatment is proving ineffectual or problematic. The resulting power struggle may lead to a clash in the discourse and jeopardize the doctor's ability to continue managing the patient authoritatively. In the next example, a compliant and knowledgeable patient challenges her doctor when her cholesterol level remains high.

Example 75 Consultation Nº 22 (Doctor: Daniel, Patient: Zenobia)

8 D: *¿Como le ha [ido?]*
How have you [been?]

9 P: *[Estuvimos] en régimen de tre– mese–, má– o meno–*
[We've] been on a diet for around three months

10 D: *Mm ya*
Mm yeah

11 P: *Para ver si ésto (colesterol) bajaba y ha baja–o bien poco a pesar de que*
To see if this (the cholesterol) would go down, and it's gone down very little despite

12 *yo hice una dieta bastante rigurosa=*
the fact that I've followed the diet quite rigorously=

13 D: *=Ya=*
=Yeah=

14 P: *=No comí huevo–, no comí mantequilla, ehm: carne– chan–, cerdo ehm:*
=I haven't had eggs, I haven't had butter, ehm: meats por–, pork ehm:,

15 *fritura– sólo verdura y fruta*
fried food I've only eaten vegetables and fruit

16 D: *¿Cuánto tenía (colesterol) ante–?*
What was your (cholesterol) level before?

17 P: *Eh: do– noventa*
Eh: two ninety

18 D: *Ya bajó a dos cincuenta=*
It's gone down to two fifty=

19 P: *=Treinta gramos. Treinta, treinta, o cuarenta.¡NAda!*
=Thirty grams. Thirty, thirty, or forty. NOthing!

20 D: *¿Cuándo se hizo Uste– el examen?=*
When did you have your last test?=

21 P: *=Ahora la semana pasada*
=Recently, last week

22 D: *No, ¿el anterior a éste?*
No, the week before?

23 P: *En el mes de junio. Junio me parece que fue y de ahí en eso estamo–. Me dieron*
In June. June I think it was, and since then it hasn't gone down. They put

24 *un régi[men]*
me on a [diet]

25 D: *[Do] noventa <WH ((lee los resultados de los examenes)) WH>*
[Two] ninety <WH ((the doctor reads the test results)) WH>

26 P: *¿Se fija? Sí, fue muy poco:=*
Can you see? It was very little:=

27 D: *=Sí, vamo– a tener que agregarle un medi[camento]*
=Yes, we'll have to increase your medic[ation]

Zenobia performed her role of competent patient by showing compliance with her low-cholesterol diet. She followed the requirements *rigurosa[mente]* ("rigorously") and avoided eating food that was contra-indicated: *huevo– ... mantequilla ... carne– ... cerdo ... fritura–* ("eggs ... butter ... meats ... pork ... fried food"). Despite this, her cholesterol level is still high. Line 9 in the example introduces the first note of possible conflict, with the patient's use of a first-person plural conjugated verb *estuvimos* ("we've"). This indicates that Zenobia now regards herself as having sufficient knowledge to be an equal player in the medical decisions made on her behalf. She issues her first challenge in line 11 when she exclaims that the cholesterol level *ha baja–o bien poco* ("has gone down very little"). The challenge becomes a complaint in line 19 when she describes the diet as useless. She raises the pitch of her voice and her talk becomes louder as she summarizes what it has achieved: *¡NAda!* ("NOthing!"). Finally, in line 26 a challenge is issued in the form of a question *¿Se fija?* ("Can you see?").

Here the *Challenger* has taken on the *voice* of the *Educator*, intruding completely into the doctor's domain! In lines 9 through to 15 Zenobia presents her own *Assessment and review* of the situation, punctuated only by Dr. Daniel's *continuer markers* in lines 10 and 13. In line 16 the doctor reasserts his *Doctor voice* with a *QSI one* and attempts to retake the floor in line 18 with his own utterance of *Assessment and review*. Zenobia's response to this, however, is scornful and dismissive, and the doctor must resort to another question in the *Doctor voice* in line 20 in order to save *face* and restore order. Rapid shifts of footing continue to the end of the passage, concluding with the doctor's *agreement marker Sí* ("Yes") and *Assessment and review* summary *vamo– a tener que agregarle un medi[camento]* ("we'll have to increase your medi[cation]"). While both participants may concur in this decision, it is also true that the authority to prescribe medications is the only power remaining to the doctor at this stage of the interview.

Zenobia's dissatisfaction with her treatment and management has put Dr. Daniel in a difficult position. The patient has certainly demonstrated compliance and competence and taken responsibility for her health. But instead of the expected rewards of personal satisfaction and improved health, her cholesterol level is not under control, and so she, too, does not feel in control. Armed with medical information about her condition, including, probably the consequences of having high cholesterol, and growing frustration, Zenobia becomes the *principal* of a text normally *authored* by the medical expert – and she is certainly the *animator* on this occasion! Now it is the doctor's competence that is under scrutiny. By shifting her alignment away from the authority of the medical institution towards that of her own knowledge, Zenobia demonstrates that a competent patient is a powerful individual. And yet, her re-presentation at the Clinic indicates that she stills seeks medical help, even if she demands careful work on Dr. Daniel's part to restore the discourse.

Because this study was confined to follow-up visits, initial-visit *Challengers* have been excluded from the analysis. These patients may contest the initial diagnosis or prescription given by the doctor on the basis of their existing background knowledge.

7.4 The *voice* of *Social Communicator*

In the course of conversation with their doctors, patients often raise issues that relate to their social identities and experiences. The central concern of both male and female patients in this study was the family. Patients referred to *mi familia* ("my family"), *mis hijos* ("my children"), *mi marido/señora* ("my husband/wife"), *mis padres* ("my parents"), *mis hermanos* ("my siblings"), *mis tías/tíos* ("my aunties/uncles") and so on, and their responsibilities as carers were apparent in the data. In this section I present two cases of the *Social Communicator*, one involving a male patient and the other a female patient.

In this first example the patient shares with the doctor the story of his father's death. The family is the focus of his attention.

Example 76 Consultation Nº 17 (Doctor: Daniel, Patient: Tito)

48 D: *¿Muy tenso en el trabajo, no está mal genio o cosa así?*
Are you very tense in your job, are you feeling irritated or something like that?

49 P: *No, lo que tuve ahora hace poco problema– familiare–*
No, but what I've had recently (are) some family problems

50 D: *Ya ¿qué le pasó?*
Yeah, what happened to you?

51 P: *El 2 de octubre falleció mi papá*
My father passed away on 2 October

52 D: *¡A[h:::!]*
A[h:::!]

53 P: *[Entonce–] eso me tiene medio=*
[So] I'm a bit=

The doctor's *QSI multiple choice* in line 48 may have been medically oriented, but the utterance was interpreted by the patient as a cue to disclose the subject of the family bereavement. He does not make this information explicit at first, however, referring to his father's death as *problema– familiare–* ("family problems"), but Dr. Daniel's further question in line 50 (*Ya ¿qué le pasó?*, "Yeah, what happened to you?") indicates that it is acceptable to bring personal problems to the medical interview. This is confirmed by the doctor's evaluative remark (Davis 1988) *¡Ah:::!* in line 52 that shows emotional reciprocity in the *Fellow Human voice*. The doctor's empathic response to Tito's story allows him to develop his narrative further:

Example 77 Consultation Nº 17 (Doctor: Daniel, Patient: Tito)

58 P: *Sí, <WH no po' WH> Uste– sabe que cuando uno se acuerda de él como que*
Yes. <WH no WH> You know that when we remember him

59 *viene (pena), pero estoy tratando de, de salir adelante, porque en este caso tan,*
we feel (the pain), but I'm trying to get over it, because in this case

60 *fue muy duro pa' mí, mi mamá porque somo–, yo soy único hijo=*
it was very hard for me, for my mother because we are, I'm the only child=

61 D: *=Ya=*
=Yeah=

Tito describes the emotional impact his father's death has had on his mother and on him as an only child. He uses his consultation time as an opportunity to express his feelings of a most profound and intimate nature. Both participants are operating within a framework that recognizes that the clinical interview is not confined to strictly physiological matters. (This point is highlighted in the "Results of Stage III: Semi-structured interview" – see below – where patients classify as a positive attribute the doctor's willingness to listen to them.)

The conversation with Dr. Daniel also reveals that the *Social Communicator* may wish to talk over events that primarily concern a third party. In our example, Tito is worried about his mother's health and treatment.

Example 78 Consultation Nº 17 (Doctor: Daniel, Patient: Tito)

62 P: *=Entonce– mi madre y yo, y madre como le digo está pero::=*
=So my mother and I, and my mother is, as I've telling you, but::=

63 D: *=Ya le ha afecta–o [mucho]*
Yeah. She's been very [affected]

64 P: *[Está]con una depre bastante: con dolore– de espalda,*
[She's] very depressed; she has a pain in her back,

65 *dolore– de hueso, de poco ánimo, dolor de cabeza que tiene entonce:– y no tengo na' <X X> y*
pain in her bones, she's been feeling low (she has) headaches, so: and I don't have anything <X X> and

66 *había pedi–o, estaba pidiendo hora pa' acá, pero le estaban dando pa'*
she asked for an appointment or she was trying to get an appointment here, but they gave her one for the

67 *media–o de de: novie:bre pa' verla pa' que le hicieran acá un chequeo o darle alguna– pastilla– a*
middle of November for a check-up or to prescribe her some medication or other

68 *tomar alguna cosa, algún relajante para no sé, pero no me pude conseguir hora acá*
a tranquillizer for I don't know what, but I couldn't make an earlier appointment

69 *así que voy a tener que ir por fuera pa' ver si::. Fue bastante duro. Sí, el se trató*
so I'll need to make one in another centre. It was very hard. Yes, he (my father) was treated

70 *aquí en la Católica, acá le trataron la enfermeda– tenía un cáncer a la próstata …*
here at the Católica (hospital). They treated him for prostate cancer …

71 *Entonce:– Fue bastante, bastante duro … (N) (Hx) …*
So: it was very, very hard … (N) (Hx) …

Here the focus is on the mother, but Tito's story also reflects the burden of responsibility he feels in caring for her. He has come to the visit as a patient with a medical problem (he is suffering from back pain and depression) and with a feeling of being a victim of circumstances (*skandalon* syndrome – Rehbein 1980, quoted in Davis 1988). He feels powerless to overcome his own medical problems and to fulfil the socio-cultural expectations upon him to look after his family, even though he expresses alignment to this role. His repetitive utterances *fue muy duro* ("it was very hard") in line 60 and *Fue bastante duro* ("It was very hard") in lines 69 and 71 emphasize this. Dr. Daniel's *helpful utterance completion* in line 63 conveys his empathy and signals that he considers it appropriate for Tito to continue talking. He may recognize that by deflecting the focus onto his mother's health and management, Tito is trying to save *face* by representing himself as someone less powerless than he feels. Examples 76–78 confirm Stivers and Heritage's finding that when patients volunteer *expanded answers* (answers that extend the minimum contribution) during the consultation, this helps the health professional to have "some degree of access to [their] life circumstances" (2001: 155).

Our second case of a *Social Communicator* is a female patient whose obligations and responsibilities are as a wife and mother of three teenage sons. From the extract we learn that she does not work outside the home, but has a number of interests, including gardening, painting and reading. For many years she has gone camping with her family during the summer holidays. In the following lines she expresses her discontent about engaging in this activity when she would rather have time for herself.

Example 79 Consultation Nº 13 (Doctor: Carlos, Patient: Olga)

303 P: *Ademá– que mi– vacacione– nunca han sido vacacione–=*
Also my holidays have never been proper holidays=

304 D: *=Ya=*
=Yeah=

305 P: *=Tengo una casa rodante=*
=I've a caravan=

306 D: *=Ya=*
=Yeah=

307 P: *=Un motor, entonce– ir a veranear*
=A caravan, so we use it to go on holidays

308 D: *No es placer para Uste–*
It's not a pleasure for you

309 P: *Eh pa' mi hijo fantástico, regio, estupendo*
Eh, for my children (it's) fantastic, superb, marvellous

310 D *[Para Uste– seguir trabajando]*
[For you, it keeps you working]

311 P: *[Aunque esté embarazada en cual]quier río lavando entonce– toda esa cosa así. Ya*
[Even when I was pregnant] I was in the lake washing– and things like that. Now

312 *estoy cansa–a pero tengo que hacerlo igual, o sea me gusta salir me gusta*
I'm tired, but I have to go anyway. I like going out

313 *yo por mí me acostara en la playa a leer un libro*
but if it were up to me, I'd lie down on the beach and read a book

314 D: *Esa serían su vacacione– ideale–*
That would be your ideal holiday

315 P: *Eso sería mis vacacione– ideal–=*
That would be my ideal holiday=

In line 303 Olga presents as a mother who sacrifices her own enjoyment by going camping even though she dislikes it. She goes because she has no choice in the matter (*tengo que hacerla igual,* "I have to go anyway") (line 312), and because she accepts that her children find the experience *fantástico, regio, es-*

tupendo ("fantastic, superb, marvellous") (line 309). For Olga, reading and relaxing on a beach would be the ideal holiday, but Dr. Carlos is unable to appreciate what she is saying.

Example 80 Consultation Nº 13 (Doctor: Carlos, Patient: Olga)

316 D: =*En un hotel donde la atienda todo, todo=*
=(You'd like to be) in an hotel where you are looked after totally, totally=

317 P: =*No, no=*
=No, no=

318 D: =*Un lugar donde la puedan atender=*
=A place where you are looked after=

319 P: =*En la casa rodante no má– pero, comer cuando quiero, cuando tengo hambre.*
=In the caravan, that's all, but (I would like) to eat when I want to, when I'm hungry

320 *Si tengo hambre, tengo. Si no, no tengo*
If I'm hungry, I eat, and if I'm not, I don't.

This exchange displays the "mismatched schema" (Tannen & Wallat 1993:70) of doctor and patient, highlighting the divergence in "participants' expectations about people, objects, events and settings in the world, as distinguished from alignment being negotiated in a particular interaction" (Tannen 1993:60). For Dr. Carlos, with his higher economic status, an ideal holiday would be a stay in an expensive hotel. It is not in his "knowledge schema" to imagine solitude in a humble caravan as a pleasurable event, nor, apparently, to recognize that luxury accomodation would be out of the question for Olga in any case. She is obliged to interrupt his train of thought in line 317 (*No, no*) and again in line 319 (*En la casa rodante no má–*, "In the caravan, that's all") to assert her position.

The conversation continues, but not with an affiliative comment by Dr. Carlos that would have supported Olga's assertion. Rather he asks a question that reveals his failure to understand her problem.

Example 81 Consultation Nº 13 (Doctor: Carlos, Patient: Olga)

321 D: *¿Por qué no puede hacerlo?*
Why can't you do it?

322 P: *Por lo– hijo– porque hay tienen hambre hay que lavar[le]*
Because of the children. I have to cook for them, do their wash[ing]

323 D: *[¿Ellos] participan?*
Do [they] help?

324 *Es cosa de hacerlo [participar]*
It's just a matter of making them [co-operate]

325 P: *[Sí este año] ello– lavaban loza ello– cooperaban con cosa que jamá–*
[Yes, this year] they washed the dishes and co-operated as never before

326 *Es que son todos seguido 14 15 13 ya este año 16 15 14=*
The fact is they were born one year apart. They're 14 15 13, and this year 16 15 14=

327 D: =*Ya*=
=Yeah=

In Chilean society, as a general rule, women are responsible for keeping the family together and raising the children, while men are usually the main income-earners. Although a modest cultural shift is occurring in Chilean society and men are gradually taking more responsibility for what has traditionally been regarded as "women's work" (Servicio Nacional de la Mujer 2003), this has not changed the social expectations placed on women. The communication breakdown here is caused by the doctor's lack of recognition of these different gender roles; as a man, he is unable to put himself in Olga's shoes.

The *voice* of *Social Communicator* exists when the medical interview provides a forum for patients to discuss personal or emotional difficulties that are impinging on their physical health. However, the extent of the doctor's empathy may be limited by a differential understanding and interpretation of the event. In Examples 76–78 Dr. Daniel was able to relate to Tito as a *Fellow Human*, as he too would undergo a sense of loss and have similar family responsibilities should his own father pass away. In Example 71, in contrast, Dr. Carlos withdrew from any engagement with Nicolás on political matters, perhaps because they were ideologically opposed. Similarly, in Dr. Carlos's consultation with Olga, the differences in the socio-economic background, gender roles and knowledge schema of each participant left little common ground for the *Fellow Human voice* to interact with the patient's story. As a consequence, Olga's *Social Communicator voice*, too, was suppressed.

7.5 The *voice* of *Initiator*

Initiators seek information about their health condition and so prompt the *Educator voice* to participate in the discourse. They project themselves as people who acknowledge that they lack the necessary knowledge to deal with their health problem, but show alignment to medical authority by calling on the doctor's expertise. *Initiators* are potential *Compliers*, since the questions they ask indicate a desire to understand more about their health in order to take better care of it.

In the example given below the questions initiated by the patient focus on understanding which kinds of foods to avoid on a cholesterol-free diet.

Example 82 Consultation Nº 21 (Doctor: Daniel, Patient: Yolanda)

122 P: *...Ahora son cosa– de de alimento, doctor, ¿las almendra–?*
... Now, doctor, I want to ask you about, about food. Almonds?

123 D: *A una persona le pueden caer mal, pero eso depende de cada persona. No hay na–a*
They're not good for some people, but that depends on the individual. There's nothing

124 P: *Pero no hay ninguna contra indicación por colesterol, [por algo]*
But there's not a contra-indication for cholesterol, [or something]

125 D: *[A Uste–]*
[For you]

126 P: *Uhm*
Mm

127 D: *Lo que sea de vegetale– o grasa– vegetale– no tiene problema: Uste– pa' eso*
You don't have any problem with vegetables or vegetable fat.

128 P: *Ya*
Yeah

129 D: *Con las grasa– animales*
But with animal fat

130 P: *¿Y el aceite de oliva?*
And olive oil?

131 D: *No, tampoco=*
No (problem), either=

132 P: *=Tampoco, ¿eh la– gelatina–?*
=Nor with jelly?

133 D: *Eh, bueno eso es agua con azúcar y colorante. No tiene mayo::r*
Eh, well, that's water with sugar and colouring. It doesn't have::

134 P: *No hay proteína–*
It doesn't have protein

135 D: *<X X>*
<X X>

136 P: *¿E– qué?*
What?

137 D: *E– químico, no tiene na–a de, no tiene na–a de alimenticio, digamo–, salvo lo– hidrato–*
Eh, (it's a) chemical. It doesn't have anything, it doesn't have anything of nutritional value, let's say

138 *de carbono de azúcar– que tienen*
except for the carbohydrates

139 P: *Uhm ya, eh y la– conserva– de marisco por ejemplo, ¿siguen siendo: eh: aunque estén*
Mm yeah, eh, and canned seafood, for example, does it keep the same nutritional

140 *en conserva siguen manteniendo lo– mismo– previsión? digo pero si es una vez*
properties, even if it's canned? I say this because sometimes once a month

141 *al mes mi marido quiere un caldillo*
my husband wants seafood soup

142 D: *Sí, no, no hay problema*
Yes, that's not a problem

143 P: *¡Ah! allí no hay problema ya*
Ah! there isn't problem with that, yeah

Yolanda initiates the episode in a forthright manner with the opening line *Ahora son cosa– de alimento, doctor* ("Now, doctor, I want to ask you about food") and proceeds with her list of specific food items. She demonstrates competence in having considered her questions in advance and compliancy in having initiated the educative episode. Dr. Daniel responds mainly in his *Educator voice* to each of her questions, and in so doing builds up the patient's knowledge and probably the effectiveness of her diet.

The sequence pattern of the *Initiator* exchange is thus one of *QSI* (asked by the patient) and answer (provided by the doctor). The *voice* of *Initiator* shares with the *voice* of *Competence* a desire to demonstrate concordance with medical advice. The *Initiator* is more assertive, however, in seeking to be empowered by knowledge.

McKenzie (2002) has noted that some patients tend to write a list of questions before visiting their doctor and are determined to get a reply – Yolanda above is a good example of this – but others believe that it is inappropriate to ask either specific questions or any questions at all and that doing so may even damage the doctor–patient relationship (Adler et al. 1998). In another study (Tran et al. 2003) a female patient had refused to ask questions because she did not want to display her ignorance; adopting the *voice* of *Initiator* was, for her, a potentially *face*-threatening act.

> On the one hand, in medical encounters, to request presupposes some determination of a candidate health problem or some level of risk for a problem; on the other hand, to request is to open the door to the awkward if not face-threatening prospect of being refused. Patients and doctors draw on resources of everyday talk to maneuvre through these dilemmas. (Gill et al. 2001: 57)

Patients less forthright than Yolanda, or less sure about the role of *Initiator* in the exchange, need helpful encouragement from their doctor to elicit this *voice*. In view of Weitzman and Weitzman's (2003) finding that the key to the success of the medical consultation is for the patient to ask questions, this does not always occur in practice.

7.6 Statistical findings

Patients' *voices* were heard, naturally enough, in all 22 of the consultations recorded for this study. Interestingly, however, while more than one *voice* was present in each consultation, no single *voice* was present in all. Table 24 summarizes the number of consultations that contained each *voice*, while Table 25 describes the total number of occurrences of each type of *voice* found in the data.

The *voice* of *Competence* (33.8%) and the *voice* of *Health-related storytelling* (30.4%) were the most frequently occurring patient *voices* during the history-taking and treatment and management routines. This is an intriguing finding in terms of the asymmetrical framework of the exchange. As we have seen, patients who come to the visit as *Health-related storytellers* delegate responsibility for their care to the institution and show alignment to the doctor's authority and power. *Competent* patients, on the other hand, are motivated to share the responsibility, and the knowledge they acquire in the process may lead to conflict with the doctor's power and authority. These two – contrasting – *voices* were almost equally balanced in the study.

We should note that although the *Social Communicator* was least represented in the data, this does not mean that it is the least important. On the contrary, when patients with difficult life issues are given an opportunity to "talk things over" with their doctor, a valuable – sometimes essential – service is provided. The *voice* of *Social Communicator* can be constrained, however, by differences in economic status and socio-cultural assumptions, and inevitable time constraints of the appointment schedule may also play a part.

The related *voices* of *Competence* and *Initiator* were explored further by analysing their frequency in the discourse of male and female patients. Table 26 shows that both females and males used the *voice* of *Competence* with similar frequency, whereas the *Initiator* was far more likely to be female, both in the number of episodes overall and in the number of individual female patients

Table 24. Patients' *voices* in the 22 consultations

Voice	Number of consultations occurring in	%
Health-related storytelling	17	77
Competence	17	77
Social Communicator	11	50
Initiator	11	50

Table 25. Patients' *voices*: total frequencies for each *voice*

Voice	Total frequency	%
Health-related storytelling	61	30.4
Competence	68	33.8
Social Communicator	34	16.9
Initiator	38	18.9
TOTAL	201	100

Table 26. *Voices* of *Competence* and *Initiator*: frequencies for female/male patients

Voice	Females	%	Males	%	Total
Competence	35	51.5	33	48.5	68
Initiator	24	63.2	14	36.8	38

who used this voice. In other words, women were usually the initiators, and initiated more often. Yolanda's repeated questioning of Dr. Daniel in Example 82 above is a good example of this. Further discussion of the important role of these two *voices* in the consultation is presented in Section 9.6 below.

The analysis also investigated possible patterns of linguistic behaviour in the gender pairings of doctors and patients. These results should be interpreted with caution, however, since other variables, such as age, experience and the nature of the illness, which may also function dynamically in the exchange, have not been isolated. The limitations of the data for gender analysis because of the higher number of female patients overall (13 out of the 22) is also freely acknowleged. Nonetheless, it may be useful to explore whether a correlation exists between the composition of the dyad and the patient's use of a particular *voice*. These findings are summarized in Table 27, and show that female patients used the *voice* of *Social Communicator* more frequently than males, accounting for 26 of the 34 episodes. However, a preference for communicating with a male or female doctor was not clear from the data. Male patients, on the other hand, were apparently more comfortable when talking about life issues with male doctors, though less likely to use this *voice* overall. In contrast to this, Dr. Ana's male patients adopted the *voice* of *Health-related storytelling* more often (13 occurrences) with her than did both Dr. Daniel's and Dr. Carlos's combined (12). In Dr. Ana's consultations with male patients, the *voice* of *Social Communicator* appears to have been suppressed by the other three *voices*, of which *Health-related storytelling* was the dominant *voice*.

The *Initiator voice* of male patients, similarly, was heard more frequently in Dr. Ana's consultations (8 occurrences) than in those of the two male doctors combined (6). Female patients, on the other hand, initiated 23 of their 24 episodes with male doctors. One female patient only asked a single question of her female doctor! The *voice* of *Competence* appears to have been fairly evenly spread across the groups.

Finally, Table 28 distributes the data for individual doctors and their patients. Dr. Ana and Dr. Carlos had the highest number of *Health-related storytelling* episodes in their consultations with both female and male patients. Importantly for the analysis, all of these patients shared the common problem of psychological distress or depression, and so it is not surprising that these individuals were least likely to display initiative or competence. It is worth pointing out here that what may start out as a follow-up visit for a medical problem can turn into an initial visit for emotional difficulties if the doctor has established sufficient rapport with the patient for the patient to feel safe enough to confide his/her innermost fears. The realization of this discourse is

Table 27. Patients' *voices* with female/male doctors

Patient *voices*	Female doctors				Male doctors				Total	
	F (n=6)		M (n=3)		F (n=7)		M (n=6)		n=22	
	N	%	N	%	N	%	N	%	N	%
Health-related storytelling	17	28	13	21	19	31	12	20	61	30.4
Competence	18	26.4	10	14.6	17	25	23	34	68	33.8
Social Communicator	14	41.1	1	2.7	12	35.2	7	12	34	16.9
Initiator	1	2.6	8	21	23	60.4	6	16	38	18.9
TOTAL	50	24.8	32	15.9	71	35.3	48	23.8	201	100

n = number of consultations
N = frequency
M = mean frequency per consultation

Table 28. Patients' *voices*: frequencies for individual doctors and female/male patients

Voice	Dr. Ana		Dr. Berta	Dr. Carlos		Dr. Daniel		Total
	F (n=3)	M (n=3)	F (n=3)	F (n=3)	M (n=3)	F (n=4)	M (n=3)	
Health-related storytelling								
N	13	13	4	12	9	7	3	61
M	4.3	14.3	1.3	4.0	3.0	1.7	1.0	29.0%
Competence								
N	6	10	12	8	12	9	11	68
M	2.0	3.3	4.0	2.6	4.0	2.2	3.6	33.8%
Social Communicator								
N	12	1	2	12	6	0	1	34
M	4.0	0.3	0.6	4.0	2.0	0.0	0.3	16.9%
Initiator								
N	1	8	0	13	6	10	0	38
M	0.3	2.6	0.0	4.3	2.0	2.5	0.0	18.9%
TOTAL	32	23	18	45	33	26	15	201 100%

only possible, of course, when doctors use the *Fellow Human voice* in response to the patient's initial *Health-related storytelling*. This was clearly the case in the exchange between Dr. Daniel and Tito in Examples 76–78.

Table 28 also shows that males used their *voice* of *Competence* more frequently with male than with female doctors, although the difference was modest. I would like to tentatively hypothesize that this finding may be related to the role of men in Chilean society more generally. In a society in which men are respected and achieve self-respect through power, the inherent power imbalance of the medical consultation places more pressure on men to save *face*, and this can be achieved to some extent by asserting their competence when confronting the doctor. For males consulting Dr. Carlos and Dr. Daniel it was also the predominant of their four *voices*. Women also used this *voice*, as we have seen, but perhaps are less bound by patriarchal imperatives to align it with their social roles. Interestingly, however, the relative use of this *voice* varied widely according to the individual doctor: for Dr. Berta's female patients it was clearly the most common voice (12 occurrences), whereas it ranked third or last with women consulting the other three doctors.

The *voice* of *Social Communicator* was the second-most common *voice* for female patients consulting both Dr. Ana and Dr. Carlos – an interesting finding in view of the gender conflict that was evident in Olga's consultation with Dr. Carlos in Example 80 above. It should be noted in this respect that two patients in particular, whose medical visit was in the nature of a counselling session in which they talked about their personal problems relating to family issues, contributed most in this *voice*.

Finally, the two groups in which the *Initiator voice* was absent altogether (Dr. Berta with females, Dr. Daniel with males) were also those in which patient *voices* were heard the least overall.

Figure 6 illustrates the functions associated with patient's *voices*.

7.7 Results of Stage III: Semi-structured interview

The semi-structured interview was performed during Stage III of this study (see Chapter 3, p. 50), with the aim of gathering patients' views on what they considered to be positive attributes of doctors. Two questions aimed at determining what patients liked (*¿qué le gusta de un médico?*, "What do you like about a doctor?") and disliked (*¿qué no le gusta de un médico?*, "What do you dislike about a doctor?") were analysed. The interviews revealed that patients

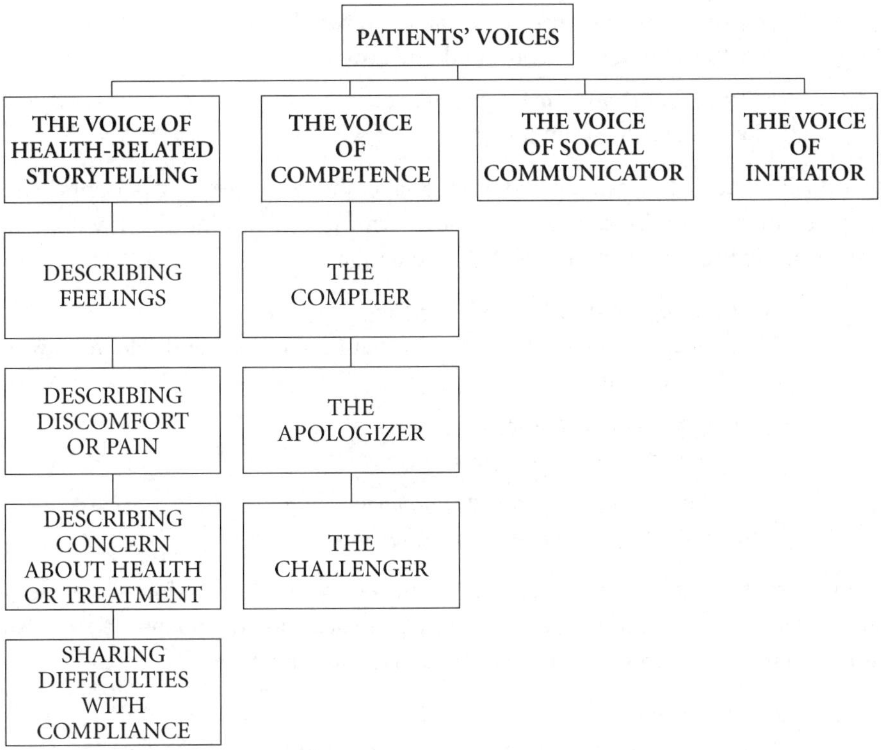

Figure 6. Discourse functions of *Patients' voices*

were very articulate in expressing their opinions, and the following four main themes emerged. Patients responded best to:

a. Sympathetic communication
b. Language that was clear and jargon-free
c. Medical and technical competence
d. Friendly and familiar communication

Sympathetic communication includes the ability to listen, to understand, and to answer questions, with respect, support, reliability, patience and optimism. It creates an atmosphere of trust and facilitates the free exchange of information (Cordella 1999: 38). Patients expressed sympathetic communication in these terms:

> *Me gusta que me escuche*
> I like a doctor who listens to me

> *Me gusta tener confianza venir con los brazos abiertos*
> I like to feel that I can come and open up to the doctor
>
> *Me gusta un médico que me entienda bien*
> I like a doctor who can understand me well

Communication in clear, everyday language shows respect to patients who may be unfamiliar with specialist medical terminology, while still allowing and encouraging them to participate in the exchange.

> *Que le explique para que uno lo entienda, sin jerga*
> [I like] doctors who explain in a way that I can understand, (doctors) who do not use jargon
>
> *Que sea claro para explicarme*
> [I like] a doctor who explains to me clearly
>
> *Que conteste a mis preguntas de una forma clara*
> [I like] a doctor who answers my questions clearly

Medical and technical competence is displayed in the thoroughness and deftness of the medical examination, a prompt and accurate diagnosis, ordering of appropriate tests, and prescribing of the correct medication.

> *Que me examine bien*
> [I like] a doctor who examines me thoroughly
>
> *Que le haga bueno examenes*
> [I like] a doctor who prescribes the right medical test to be carried out

Finally, patients liked doctors who were not only skilful in their medical work and professional in their conduct, but were also able to communicate in a friendly, warm and affectionate manner so that the exchange felt more like a conversation between friends.

> *Me gusta cuando el médico es abierto para contarle penas y dolores*
> I like it when my doctor and I can have a heart-to-heart.

Even though patients seek help from, and mostly align to, medical authority, they do not like doctors who display a sense of superiority. Instead, a familiar and less asymmetrical interaction is preferred.

> *Que no sea un médico estirado. Uno sabe que ellos saben, pero no me gusta que me lo muestren*
> [I like] a doctor who is not snob. I know that they are knowledgeable, but I don't like them to demonstrate that to me

Que no sea hosco. Soy el doctor, soy Dios
[I like] a doctor who is not surly. "I'm the doctor, I'm God".

In summary, patients seek professional and competent doctors who are able to treat their health problem as quickly and as simply as possible. However, once the doctor's superior knowledge and power have been tacitly acknowledged, patients want to feel that their doctors relate to them as *people*. The rapport that is created in the exchange appears to be of vital importance: "indeed, three of the four categories [are] related to the rapport created in the exchange between the doctor and the patient" (Cordella 1999: 39).

The opinions of female and male patients recorded in the semi-structured interview are summarized in Table 29. Sympathetic communication was nominated as an important aspect of doctor's behaviour 89 times, ahead of medical and technical competence (50 times), while the other two attributes scored 32 and 28 counts respectively. Sympathetic communication was the most recorded attribute of both men and women, but almost one-half of the males listed medical and technical competence compared with just over one-third of females. While patients were not asked to rank the attributes, the raw data suggests nonetheless that when anxious or unwell people (of either sex) entrust their health to a medical professional, the thing they value most is a safe and reassuring environment in which to talk about their problems. Indeed, a sympathetic ear may be the battle half won.

7.8 Conclusion

This chapter has shown that patients may use a range of *voices* in the course of the consultation that not only provide factual information related to their health problem but also indicate levels of competence and compliance. These *voices* may be initiated by the patient spontaneously or prompted by the doctor's questioning; their presence or absence can be an indicator of the patient's passive or active role in the exchange. Doctors give patients the opportunity to take the floor and facilitate their talk through use of the *Fellow Human voice*, while patients take the opportunity provided by the consultative setting to talk about their illness, their health management, and their daily lives.

We have also seen that these patients' *voices* do not always dovetail with doctors' *voices*, and that this can lead to conflict. The *voice* of *Competence*, in particular, has been shown to be problematic: on the one hand, competence is a sign of the patient's awareness, sense of responsibility and compliance with

Table 29. Positive attributes of doctors' communication: nominations by female/male patients

Attribute	Female patients (94 interviewees*)		Male patients (33 interviewees**)		Total	%
	N	%	N	%		
Sympathetic communication	70	46.1	19	40.4	89	44.8
Language that is clear and jargon-free	25	16.4	7	14.9	32	16.1
Medical and technical competence	35	23.0	15	31.9	50	25.1
Friendly communication	22	14.5	6	12.8	28	14.0
TOTAL	152	76.4	47	23.6	199 ***	100

* I distributed questionnaires to 96 patients, but two did not answer which doctor attribute(s) they considered positive.

** 38 male patients received the questionnaire, but 5 failed to answer these questions.

*** Because some patients mentioned more than one attribute in their response, the total is greater than the number of interviewees.

medical recommendations; on the other, competence can lead to a shift in footing and challenges to the doctor's authority. The final two chapters will explore the dynamic relationship between doctors' and patients' voices, and the concepts of asymmetry, power and affiliative discourse styles will be brought to bear on the results.

Note

1. On 11 September 1973 the military overthrew the democratically elected government of Salvador Allende and assumed power.

Chapter 8

Patterns of footing

Section 2.1.1 outlined Goffman's (1963, 1971, 1981, 1983) framework of interaction as it concerns the shifts in alignment or stance (*footing*) of participants in the discourse. In this brief chapter I want to explore some of the patterns of footing that emerged in the data, and to argue that a shift from one *voice* to another corresponds to a re-balancing of the interaction between doctor and patient, and that by continual shifting and re-balancing the consultation becomes dynamic.

Firstly, let us look at how the *Educator voice* functions in the talk by identifying the discourse patterns that favour the appearance and development of this alignment in the exchange. This *voice* is especially relevant in the present study, since the research was undertaken in a teaching hospital where one would expect attention to education to be paramount.

The data shows that the doctor may either initiate the educative episode spontaneously (usually after reading the patient's test results) or after the patient, as *Initiator*, has asked for some information. These two ways of introducing the *Educator voice* were the most prevalent in the 15 conversations where this *voice* was present (cf. asterisked value in Table 15, p. 115). The length of time and the number of turns spent in this *voice* will depend on the topic being discussed as well as on other variables affecting the discourse. Thus, the doctor may have one or more turns in one *voice* before shifting to another *voice* where the number of turns may vary again. In what follows I present the main patterns of the *Educator voice* found in this study.

Given the patient's presentation primarily for medical care, we would expect to find the most common shifts occurring from *Doctor voice* (D) to *Educator voice* (E) (via one of the patient's (P) *voices*) and vice versa. When the *Doctor voice* initiates the episode it is typically engaged in one of two types of discourse associated with follow-up visits, namely (a) Assessment of test results, or (b) Assessment of patient compliance. The *Educator voice* that follows the *Doctor voice* is engaged in either (a) Communicating medical facts, or (b) Communicating medical treatment and management. Usually this discourse pattern comes to an end when the doctor seeks further information from the patient, which, as we saw in Chapter 4, was the most common function of the *Doctor voice*. This *three-step* footing pattern is summarized in Figure 7.

D → (P) → E → (P) → D

Figure 7. Discourse pattern *Doctor – Educator – Doctor*

In this pattern, the *Doctor voice* initiates the discourse followed by the *Educator voice*. The patient may respond to the *Educator voice*, or the doctor may end the episode and initiate a question in the *Doctor voice* in the same utterance.

The second discourse pattern is associated with the patient's *Initiator voice* (I). Patients ask questions that relate to medical issues and this prompts the doctor to respond as *Educator*. Here doctors *author* and *animate* a voice of authority as they explain the medical matter at hand. The end of the *Educator voice* is again usually marked by the doctor's shift to the *Doctor voice*; this new footing may seek additional information from the patient with a view to developing another educative episode building on the first, or perhaps to take the discourse in a new direction. This *three-step* footing pattern is represented in Figure 8.

I → E → (P) → D

Figure 8. Discourse pattern *Initiator – Educator – Doctor*

The pattern I → E can be extended for as long as the patient continues to ask questions and the doctor is willing to answer them. This means that the number of turns of the *Educator voice* may be as much a factor of the patient's recurrent questioning (Example 82 is a good example of this) as it is of the doctor's own initiative in introducing the educative episode.

The performance of patients' *voices* and their shift from one *voice* to another were also investigated in this study. It was found that patients' footing is partly, but not entirely, conditioned by doctor *voices*, and that patients do not always present a predictable linguistic pattern in medical discourse. In order to clarify these findings I start by presenting two common relationships.

The *voice* of *Health-related storytelling* (HSt) is most commonly associated with the *Doctor voice*: that is, doctors seek information about their patients' health, and patients give an account of their condition (Examples 70, 71). The *voice* of *Competence* (C), too, pairs with the *Doctor voice* in its second function of assessment and review: the doctor wishes to determine the extent of the patient's understanding and compliance with medical recommendations, and the patient replies in one of the *voices* of *Competence* (Examples 72–74). The sequence generally concludes with a return to the *Doctor voice*. This is summarized in Figure 9.

D → HSt or C → D

Figure 9. Discourse pattern *Doctor – Health-related storytelling / Competence – Doctor*

There were a few examples in the data where the third turn was taken by the *Educator voice*, but this did not prevent the patient from continuing in the *voice* of *Health-related storytelling*. Nor did the number of turns in this *voice* appear to be more a factor of the doctor's use of *QSI* and the frequency of continuer markers in the *Fellow Human voice* (FH) than of patients' individual projection of themselves (see Example 79). Figure 10 illustrates this finding.

D → HSt → [E] → HSt → [D and/or FH and/or E]

Figure 10. Discourse pattern Doctor *voices – voice* of *Health-related storytelling*

Of the 17 (out of 22) consultations in which the *voice* of *Competence* was present, patients presented a pattern of offering more than one turn related to their competence (e.g. Example 73). This was made possible by either (a) the doctor's use of CMs after each utterance, (b) the doctor's next turn taking the form of a question (e.g. Example 74) to which the patient again replied in the *voice* of *Competence*, or (c) affiliative discourse markers in the *Fellow Human voice* to prompt the patient's shift of footing to the *voice* of *Initiator*. This is illustrated as follows:

D → C → FH or D → C or FH → I

Figure 11. Discourse patterns of Doctor *voices* and the *voice* of *Competence*

The *voice* of *Social Communicator* (SC), in which the whole person of the patient is expressed in the patient's story, and the *voice* of *Initiator*, through which the patient demonstrates power and competence in the exchange, were, perhaps not surprisingly, the least likely to conform to a predictable pattern. As described above, using the *voice* of *Initiator* the patient *acts* and the doctor, as

Educator, reacts. Thus, because the *Initiator* is not predicated on a doctor *voice*, but rather the other way round, it may jump in at any point in the discourse. A patient may ask a question regardless of the doctor's current footing, and may shift to and from this *voice* at will. The presence of the *Social Communicator* may indicate that the doctor has adopted a holistic approach (i.e. both bio-medical and socio-relational) to the consultation by encouraging the patient's human story, though this is not always the case. Patients may shift to this footing with or without the assistance of the *Fellow Human voice*, and may even interpret a *Doctor voice QSI* as a cue to continue the account. Thus it is possible to find a three-part sequence initiated by either the *Doctor* or *Fellow Human* followed by the *Social Communicator* or *Initiator* and concluded by any one of *Doctor*, *Educator* or *Fellow Human*. This is set out in Figure 12.

D or FH → SC and/or I → D and/or E or FH

Figure 12. Discourse pattern Doctor *voices – voice* of *Social Communicator / Initiator*

In summary, doctors' *voices* appear to be much more prescribed than their patients', since these have been *learned* through many years of medical training and must also show alignment to their profession. Patients' voices, on the other hand, are those of untrained, non-institutional individuals and as a consequence occur with less predictability in the discourse. While some clear patterns emerge, it is also evident that each of the four patient *voices* has the potential to disrupt these patterns. The *voices* of *Health-related storytelling* and *Competence* tend to be elicited by the *Doctor voice*, but may also insist on further turns without explicit encouragement. Nor did the *Doctor voice* in my study call forth these two *voices* only. The *Initiator* may take the floor at any time, sometimes with a long list of questions (as in Example 82), or interrupt any other *voice*. The contribution of the *Social Communicator* may be modified by the presence or absence of the *Fellow Human voice*, but is not entirely dependent on it.

From this we can see that although doctors may ultimately control the discourse, since they are required to use their professional *voices* to fulfil their responsibilities as care providers, patients are not left short of options. Indeed, they are perhaps more at liberty to introduce abrupt shifts of footing, to resist efforts at shifting their footing, and to withhold one or more of their *voices*. It is the doctor's task to elicit the necessary medical information from the patient while respecting and balancing all the patient *voices* that are expressed in the exchange.

Chapter 9

The Dynamic Consultation

It is not unusual to hear complaints about the medical system and in particular about those unsuccessful consultations that patients so vividly remember. These stories are shared with friends, who contribute many more stories of their own. In Chile, for example, dissatisfaction with the public health system is almost a way of life. Martinic (1996: 2) argues that

> *En . . . Chile es ya una constante histórica la crítica que los usuarios hacen al "mal trato" que reciben por parte de los servicios públicos de salud. Esta se verbaliza como mala atención, burocracia, falta de consideración y respeto . . .*
>
> In . . . Chile, criticism of the public health system is an historical phenomenon for those who use this service and receive "ill treatment" that is verbalized as poor service, bureaucracy, absence of consideration and lack of respect . . .

Disappointment with the medical consultation has been frequently reported in medical and linguistic studies. Dawson et al. (2000: 64) indicate that Australian women from migrant communities, including Chilean, had

> Many complaints about the care they received from their doctors and they held positive opinions about the ways in which complementary medicine practioners are able to deal more adequately with "the whole person" . . . Women consider alternative medicines and the practitioners, such as Chinese medicine and homeopathy, as being more in tune with their health as a totality.

These same studies have shown that patients' opinions are based very much on their sense of the quality of the verbal exchange. Poor communication throughout the consultation, albeit subjectively defined, leaves the patient dissatisfied even if the actual medical treatment has been delivered efficiently. It behoves us, therefore, to undertake a more rigorous and objective analysis of doctor–patient discourse if we are to understand what causes these breakdowns in communication, and to identify the functional constraints that lead to a disappointing outcome.

This study focused on the contribution of both participants in the medical consultation, and by deconstructing the discourse it became clear that doctors and patients perform a set of *voices*. These *voices*, firstly, are associated with the institutional "roles" of doctor and patient, and the micro-realization of the discourse helped us to understand the interaction between doctors and patients more generally. Secondly, it was shown that these *voices* may also (re)formulate discourses found in other, socio-cultural contexts. The interconnection of these several identities will be developed further below.

9.1 Doctors' and patients' talk: *Animator, author, principal*

9.1.1 *Doctor voice* and *Educator voice*

The *voices* of doctors and patients, as they have been defined and identified in this study, are markers of each participant's role in the consultation, alignment to medical authority, and social status (Fairclough 1989: 46). Use of these *voices* is to some extent a function of these markers, but may also be a function of the individual's personality or the nature of the medical problem.

Following Goffman (1981: 167), both doctor and patient act as *animators* in the exchange, through their respective contributions to the discourse. We have identified a number of similarities in their talk: for example, each may ask questions, seek information, use agreement discourse markers, remain silent, and so on. The data also showed that doctors and patients in this study used a remarkably similar number of words overall (see Section 3.13). As *animators*, therefore, their participation was comparable in the exchange.

Doctors and patients also take their turn as *authors* and *principals*, but here the asymmetry in their roles becomes evident. When using the *Doctor voice* or *Educator voice*, doctors are duty-bound to align to the script that has been *authored* by the medical profession. It is, indeed, a critical part of their medical training to learn that script. Then, having undergone this training and chosen to enter the profession, it can be assumed that they are *principals* of that script in their utterances; that is, the information they provide and the opinions they express are believed to be true from both a personal and a professional standpoint. It may sometimes happen that the doctor's personal and professional views come into conflict; however, there was no evidence of this in the data recorded for this study.

Patients, too, act as *authors* and *principals*, but of a different script. As we have noted, theirs is an unlearned "role", and accordingly their text is informal and unrehearsed. We have also noted that when patients presume to *author* a medical text, this can be interpreted as an intrusion into the doctor's territory, an unwelcome crossing of the line. Thus, patients' scripts describe their medical problem and their understanding of it, their compliance, personal issues affecting their life, and sometimes their sense of helplessness and fear. As *author* of their own life story, they will also be, naturally enough (unless psychologically disturbed or deliberately deceitful) its *principal.*

The framework of the medical consultation operates therefore to both facilitate and limit doctors' and patients' talk in different ways. Doctors are required to adhere to orthodox bio-medical views and are not at liberty to express personal opinions that conflict with these; at the same time, the authority that comes with their expertise and their alignment with the institution of medicine gives them considerable power. Patients, on the other hand, may converse freely, but the subject of their talk is confined to matters affecting themselves; and as these generally concern some form of breakdown in their normal functioning, for which they seek help, they are at a situational disadvantage which contributes to further the asymmetry of the exchange.

9.1.2 *Fellow Human voice*

The *Fellow Human voice* allows the doctor to get closer to the patient's life-world than do either the *Doctor* or *Educator* voices. Utterances in the *Fellow Human voice* have not been formulated in medical texts; they are thus free of the specialized terminology that can act as a communication barrier in the discourse, and the subject matter is not recycled from a memorized and unassailable source, but can be of a general nature as it relates directly or indirectly to the patient's concerns. As its name suggests, therefore, this *voice* allows doctor and patient to communicate more nearly as equals. Clearly, then, the presence or absence of this *voice* when communicating with the patient is a significant choice.

The *Fellow Human voice* assimilates some of the characteristics that have been reported in the talk of other health professionals, such as female nurses. Fisher noted, when comparing medical sessions carried out by female nurses and male doctors, that female patients received a more comprehensive consultation from female nurses, who "encouraged [their patients] to talk about the social/bibliographical context of their lives – [i.e.] speak their emotions" (1995: 179). In contrast, male doctors tended to dismiss any emotional or extra-medical utterances as irrelevant. Haberland and Mey also contribute to the idea that nurses tend to fill the communication gaps left by doctors. They describe this situation as follows:

> The common situation on hospital rounds, where the nurses afterwards have to "translate" the doctor's wording of the cases into normal, understandable language, so that the patient may get an idea of their situation, is the rule rather than the exception in therapeutic communication. (1981:106)

In other words, the doctors in Haberland and Mey's study were often unable to adapt to the patient's needs by constructing a discourse that was comfortable for the patient and that would narrow the gap between them. Similarly, Fisher found that doctors tended to overlook the socio-relational side of patient care, delegating this responsibility to other health professionals. Nurses not only made more space in the discourse for patients to recount their stories, but preferred this type of conversation:

> Where the doctor provides very little space for the patient to explain what [their] symptoms mean in the context of [their] life, the nurse practioner, by asking open-ended questions, maximizes this kind of space. Where the doctor lets contextual cues pass unexplored, it is just the social clues that the nurse practioner pursues. (1991:166)

This division of responsibilities in the medical system – that is, where on the one hand there is the "curer" who treats the medical condition and on the other there is the "carer" who listens to and encourages the patient's self-expression – has been considered by Bamberg. He writes:

> Recent trends toward an increasing specialization and the necessity of an increasing technical expertise are viewed as contributing to a decrease in emphasis on the person as a whole, in particular, as one who is functioning and doing (relatively) well in his or her social and cultural life-world. Whatever may have "caused" these changes in perspectives, the common split between curing as the basic obligation of medical experts, and caring as a secondary obligation, which is handed over more and more to other caretaking professionals (nurses, social workers, psychologists, priests), seems to be widely shared in Western societies by laypeople and medical experts. (1991:330)

This separation of "basic" and "secondary" obligations was not a feature of my study, perhaps because the four doctors were general practitioners rather than specialist physicians and surgeons. We have seen in the preceding chapters that doctors used both bio-medical and socio-relational approaches with their patients, albeit to varying degrees, in the consultations. Although the medical voice projected through the *Doctor voice* was prominent when asking questions (93.98% of *QSI* compared with 6.02% in the *Fellow Human voice*), it must be remembered that questioning is only one of several affiliative discourse forms employed to show empathy.

While doctors will inevitably develop more personal rapport with some patients than others, use of the *Fellow Human voice* is part of the doctor's professional role and responsibility to care for the patient, and not an expression of personal likes and dislikes. Limitations of its use will nonetheless occur if the diverse socio-cultural backgrounds of the participants make it very difficult to establish any real connection, as was clear in Dr. Carlos's miserable attempt at social conversation with Olga in Examples 80 and 81. Put simply, doctors and patients may have very little in common. While one patient stated, "I like a doctor who can understand me well" (p. 180), it may not be easy for her doctor to appreciate her socio-economic circumstances, her interests or her lifestyle. Clearly, then, the more training doctors have in the use of this *voice*, the more satisfying the encounter will be for the patient.

9.1.3 The *voices* of *patients' stories*

In Chapter 7 we explored the idea that patients develop their stories using the *voices* of *Health-related storytelling* and *Social communicator*. Labov and Fanshel (1977) and Davis (1988) have suggested that it is the "reportability" of events that determines whether they will be recounted in future discourse; that is, they are thought to contain something that is funny, amazing, fascinating, fantastic or peculiar, something that justifies "holding the listener's attention" (Labov & Fanshel 1977: 105). Patients' stories in the present study, however, were rarely "reportable" in this sense; the most important thing for patients seemed to be the sense that they were being *listened* to, that they could recount their physical symptoms, their dreams, fears, their work/family/social concerns. As we saw in the semi-structured interview (pp. 179–182), patients rated positively doctors who allowed time to hear them and favoured a communication style that was sympathetic and intimate (*me gusta cuando el médico es abierto para contarle penas y dolores*, "I like it when my doctor and I can have a heart-to-heart"; *me gusta [un médico] que me escuche*, "I like a doctor who listens to me"). Cordella (1999) also found that patients liked doctors who were friendly, warm, affectionate, kind and pleasant when talking to them. The different findings in my study compared with those of Labov and Fanshel (1977) and Davis (1988) may perhaps be explained by different socio-cultural expectations, the context in which the conversation took place (Gumperz 1982b), and/or the particular relationship between participants in the consultation.

Of course, patients can also choose to say as little as possible, as was demonstrated by Wilma's unresponsiveness to Dr. Daniel in Example 69, or to limit their number of *voices*. Reportability may then have less to do with the worthiness of the report as such than with the patient's willingness to share it. This may be due to a number of factors, including different understandings of the participatory framework, the absence of the *Fellow Human voice*, or the inability of this *voice* to develop a rapport with the patient, for whatever reason.

The use of both the *voice* of *Social Communicator* and the *Fellow Human voice* in the discourse can be interpreted through Goffman's (1983: 11) observation that

> We quite routinely ritualise participation frameworks; that is, we self-consciously transplant the participation arrangement that is natural in one social situation into an interactional environment in which it isn't. In linguistic terms, we not only embed utterances, we embed interaction arrangements.

Thus, the "participation arrangement" of familiar conversation is transplanted to the "interactional environment" of the medical interview, but with a number of inherent asymmetries that can make the latter seem "unnatural". Both doctors and patients need to undertake the careful negotiation between "friendliness" and "friendship" in order for the consultation to be successful, and to recognize the different "roles" that are required to achieve this. Because patients often present to the medical interview at their most vulnerable or fearful, and are sometimes lonely and in need of friendship as well, this negotiation can be very delicate indeed.

Finally, it is noted that the patient's *Initiator voice* also contributes to the story by asking questions that introduce new topics of conversation to be developed.

In summary then, patients have greater freedom as *authors*, *animators* and *principals* of their utterances and as the central subject of the interview, but lack any real authority in the exchange; doctors are imbued with the power and authority that comes with their expertise and institutional position, but are restricted to their roles as *animators*, *authors* and *principals* of medical information by protocols that do not allow for the expression of personal views *per se*. On this last point, however, it should be noted that in practice, of course, doctors' personal views may infiltrate the medical discourse, particularly if these are strongly held. Accordingly, "there exists not *one* discourse in the institution, but a whole set of interwoven, conflicting discourses which construct and establish multiple relationships" (Wodak's emphasis, 1996: 12). We have identified a number of ways in which these relationships may be not only multi-layered but multiply asymmetrical.

9.2 Asymmetry, power and the use of *voices*

In this study asymmetry in the medical context was observed at two main levels: both in institutional practice and in the discourse of doctors and patients. Although my main interest was on the latter, I will introduce this section by looking briefly at the effect of institutional power on participants.

9.2.1 Asymmetry in the institution

As mentioned in Chapter 3, patients who attended the Clinic were familiar with the Medical Centre, since they had visited it before or had had carried out most of their prescribed tests there; some patients had also consulted other health professionals in the same Centre. This familiarity with the institution correlated with the amount of information kept on the patient, which was stored in personal files available in the Centre. This record-keeping may be thought of as exercising some degree of control over patients. Foucault (1980) uses the metaphor of the *Panopticon* (a circular system of gaols devised in the 19th century to better control criminals) to describe this sort of control. "Panoptism" is the material expression of surveillance and control exerted by a superior social body (such as a the state medical institution) over individuals (such as patients) through the accumulation of dossiers, records and other forms of identification. Documents are not generally available to the person but are held by, and become resources of, the institution. The interpretation of asymmetry in discourse analytical studies has been based on the unequal opportunities given to individuals and institutions to access resources (Fairclough 1989, 1992; Giddens 1976, 1977, 1987; van Dijk 1995a, 1995b, 1997b). This inequality is aggravated in settings such as a medical clinic where the person in need of the resources (the unwell patient) is the one without access to them, except through the conduit of the (presumably) healthy, well-provided doctor, who is paid to supply those resources. This situation was certainly found to be true in my study.

9.2.2 Asymmetrical questioning

The *voices* that we have identified in this book have been clearly demarcated as belonging to either doctor or patient, and we have discussed the reasons why a doctor may not adopt a patient *voice* and vice versa. Even the *Doctor voice* and *Initiator voice*, which both seek information about the patient's health, can be shown to contribute to the asymmetry of the exchange. Doctors in this study initiated the majority of the questions (356, see Table 8) compared to only 38 asked by patients (Table 26). Ainsworth-Vaughn (1994), Coulthard and Ashby (1975) and West (1984) reported similar findings in their studies, and Frankel (1984) and Ten Have (1991) reached the same conclusion after reviewing the abundant literature on questions in medical discourse. Wodak (1996: 170) argues that

> Doctors exercise power over their patients, they ask the questions, they interrupt and introduce new topics, and they control the conversation. Patients are expected to comply with the explicit and implicit norms of the clinic procedures.

In my study I have interpreted the doctor's frequent questioning as a discourse strategy to implicitly exercise control while explicitly investigating the patient's health condition. In general, the expectations put on patients to comply with this approach were realized, with a strong tendency for patients to respond to the medically oriented *Doctor voice*. However, as was noted in Section 4.1, the form of questioning determined the quality of the reply. Whereas a *QSI one* was likely to be answered with information that was sought by the doctor, a *QSI chain* or *QSI multiple choice* were less effective and could even be counter-productive, as patients were inclined to answer only one or part of the questions. In a study carried out by Hein and Wodak it was found that open questions gave patients the opportunity to "produce a self-structured reply [and to] tell a real story" (1987: 53), but they also found that a relationship existed between the types of questions asked and the level of education of the patients. Poor questioning may reflect a lack of skill on the part of the doctor, which, in the worst cases can lead to misdiagnosis because of the inadequacy of the information provided (Cicourel 1999: 183), but insistent or random questioning may also be used to exercise power in the discourse by confusing or silencing the patient's contribution.

Doctors in my study also used a greater variety of questions than their patients, with patients' questions restricted to the equivalent form of doctors' *QSI one*. Erzinger suggests that the difference between doctors' and patients' questioning is based on the different roles and responsibilities of each participant in the discourse, and that the reluctance of patients to ask questions is a positive attribute of respect for the doctor's role:

> Doctors have a prominent position as initiators in the medical encounter because their status as interviewers makes them responsible for the introduction of new topics. Spanish-speaking patients in this study maintained their re-

spectful position as good patients and initiated topics less frequently than doctors. (1989: 199)

It can be argued, however, that respect is also a form of compliance with the uncontested exercise of power in an interaction in which each participant's role is clearly allocated and their behaviour relatively fixed, regardless of the interaction that develops. Consequently, the chances of *dialectic of control* (Giddens 1984) and the freedom of participants' actions may be diminished. In any case, data supporting Erzinger's interpretation of respect did not feature strongly in my study. Rather, the ability of participants to intervene in the discourse and to alter its course (Giddens 1976: 11) was in evidence. This idea of participants as actors in the discourse will be further developed below.

9.2.3 Asymmetrical disapproval

In my data it was also possible to observe asymmetrical behaviour in the use of silence and reproving utterances. It will be recalled from Section 4.2 that one of the functions of the *Doctor voice* is to appraise whether the patient has followed medical recommendations, and that doctors' responses will vary depending on whether they are dealing with complying or non-complying patients. While doctors congratulated compliant patients for having followed the treatment as prescribed, non-compliance (understood as failure to align with medical authority) was often met with silence or implied reprimand, as we saw in Examples 19–22 (see also Cordella in press). Patients responded to doctors with silence or minimal utterances too at times (such as Wilma in Example 69) and in certain situations these may also be interpreted as discourse strategies to express displeasure. Indeed, non-compliance itself may be a manifestation of the patient's disapproval of the medical treatment or the doctor's personal style. What makes this reproachful behaviour asymmetrical, however, is that whether it is the doctor or patient who withdraws from the speech, it is ultimately the patient who is disadvantaged.

The consultation in Examples 19–22 presents an interesting scenario for looking further at the relationship between communication and compliance. It will be recalled that Hilda is telling Dr. Berta about her compliance with a weight-loss diet, but has so far failed to lose weight. Hilda's account in the *voice* of *Competence* gives Dr. Berta many opportunities to respond with affiliative utterances in the *Fellow Human voice* or to take up some of her comments and develop them using the *Educator voice*, but her next turn is always a *QSI one* in the *Doctor voice*, a silence, or an implied reproach (lines 68–69). She not only does not acknowledge Hilda's statements of compliance, thereby diminishing the chances of developing a rapport with her patient and perhaps teasing out more information that will help with the diagnosis, but also offers her no educative advice that might contribute to a better understanding of her diet.

Against this, however, we do not know the history of Dr. Berta's and Hilda's relationship. The doctor may be aware that her patient's story is not entirely truthful, and may have heard it many times before. Encouragement and empathy using the *Fellow Human voice* may have been tried and failed. A cold and negative response could in fact be a strategy to see if Hilda will respond better to an aloof and authoritarian style. The skill required of doctors is to able "read" their patients sufficiently well to know whether the stick or carrot is likely to be the most effective. While patients generally speak in favour of, and respond best to, empathy in medical encounters, this study has emphasized the dynamic role of patients' participation, and this may include (regrettably, if understandably) a reluctance in some cases to shift from a powerless position to one of greater personal responsibility. In other words, any one of the doctor's *voices* may be the appropriate *voice* to achieve compliance in a specific situation.

9.2.4 Asymmetrical knowledge

Many studies have highlighted the counter-productivity of strategies that maintain the differential knowledge of expert and layperson (Cicourel 1999; Davis 1988; Fisher 1995; Fisher & Todd 1986b; Hein & Wodak 1987; Todd & Fisher 1993; Wodak 1996).

In Chapter 5 we saw that the *Educator voice* communicates medical facts and proposes treatment to make patients more aware of the need for compliance with the management of their health condition, but in Chapter 7 we also saw that a "too-effective" education may lead to patients acquiring enough expertise to become *Challengers* (Section 7.3.3), threatening to undermine the *Doctor* and *Educator voices* and go beyond the bounds of their role. In order to maintain the status quo, therefore, it is important for the institution to uphold the distinction between educator and educated, and for ownership of knowledge as an expression of power and control always to be divided asymmetrically in the doctor's favour.

Helman (1994: 101) discusses the "enculturation" of doctors, a process through which they acquire not only medical training but also the belief that their profession is one of "high social status, high earning power and the socially legitimated role of healers, which carries with it certain rights and obligations". Wodak (1996) writes of the medical training young doctors receive:

"owing to the values and myths of the institution, they are expected to live up to the image of omniscience, although they are actually in training". According to Cicourel (1999: 190), because of the selection procedures they go through in order to be admitted into medicine, "medical students are accorded a status that other graduate or professional students seldom enjoy, and this selectivity provides an initial kind of 'aura' or charisma and power to these individuals". This situation is similar in Chile, where students must be at the upper percentile of scores in the national entry university test *Prueba de Selección Universitaria* in order to study medicine.[1]

In Examples 50 and 51 we observed the doctor "educating" the patient to respect "the gulfs that separate insiders from outsiders" (Wodak 1996: 2) by disregarding any comment on medical issues not made by a qualified health professional. A clear distinction was made between "insiders" who have all the authority and "outsiders" who have no medical credibility at all. The educative episode was triggered by the patient offering information that came from an "outside" source, causing the doctor to exclaim *Aquí en Chile lamentablemente somo– todo– potenciale– médico–* ("Unfortunately, here in Chile we are all potential doctors"). Institutional self-justification may therefore permeate the educative episodes of medical discourse and serve to promote doctors' opinions. As Fairclough and Wodak put it (1997: 258):

> Discursive practices may have major ideological effects: that is, they can help produce and reproduce unequal power relations . . . through the ways in which they represent things and position people.

If Chilean doctors really are concerned that their authority is being undermined by populist therapies, this may go part of the way towards explaining why only 15 consultations in the study included an episode in the *Educator voice*. Unfortunately, in seeking to maintain the asymmetry of knowledge in the relationship, doctors impose limits on their potential role as educators and may even jeopardise a comprehensive understanding of their patient's health. In addition, they may also lose a valuable opportunity to learn something from their patients by remaining so conservative in their views!

The use of the *Educator voice* in the function of *Responding to patient discomfort* was shown to be particularly problematic when it came to ownership of knowledge. In Example 35 the doctor deflected responsibility for the patient's headaches away from the change in medicine towards a strongly psychosomatic explanation. Example 36 showed the doctor reaffirming the medical view that tests were not necessary in spite of the patient's recurrent discomfort. In each case, the patient's own "knowledge" was interpreted as a threat rather than a helpful contribution, and consequently discounted in favour of an outcome that would save both the doctor's own *face* and also shield the reputation of the institution. Indeed, it became clear that saving a colleague's *face* or saving one's own amounted to much the same thing: both actions served the higher purpose of safeguarding the profession against charges of malpractice or incompetence, and ensuring that it spoke with one voice. My analysis has shown that doctors play a large part in maintaining the standards of the institution by undertaking surveillance and control measures in their consultations with individual patients.

Examples 35 and 36 also showed that patients deferred to doctors' superior knowledge to such an extent that they appeared to accept the doctor's interpretation of their symptoms even when this constituted a denial of their own reality. *Factual* explanations were never contested by patients in this study. Nonetheless, we have also seen patients in a less submissive role throughout this book, particularly when they bring to the discourse social responsibilities that clash with medical recommendations. The extent to which patients will allow their daily routines to be disrupted by medical treatment will depend to a large extent on the severity of the illness.

Example 48 presented a case of *selective* education. We will recall that Dr. Carlos is discussing the prospect of surgery with Olga who is suffering from pain in her arm. Dr. Carlos's manner is friendly enough, but we noted that despite her misgivings he is prepared to describe only the form of treatment that aligns with his expertise. The educative episode is therefore unbalanced in failing to address all the available possibilities for solving the patient's problem. As Fairclough writes (1989:65):

> The exercise of power: constraints on contents, subjects, and relations. In terms of the contents, discourse in a formal situation is subject to exceptional constraints on topic on relevance, and in terms of more or less fixed interactive routines.

In refusing to entertain any options other than his own "fixed interactive routine" of recommending surgery, and denying the possible value of alternative treatments, Dr. Carlos exercises power over his patient and perpetuates the asymmetry of the exchange.

9.3 Knowledge, power and *simpatía*

Consultations that require the doctor to negotiate treatment and management with the patient also require the doctors' *voices* to respond dynamically, or as Holmes et al. put it (1999: 377), "superiors in the workplace 'do power' in interactions in a variety of ways". Wodak (1996: 47) found that the doctor's manner may range "from a gentle approach through stiff formality and impatience to harsh authority" and, similarly, Davis (1988: 107) describes the

> Occasional instance of ... straightforward, authoritarian control ... [as] by far, the exception. Rather than being characterized by coercion or restraint, the most pervasive feature of my consultations was a quality of friendly intimacy. They bore more resemblance to a chat between friends than a chilly institutional encounter headed by a harsh, authoritarian physician.

Doctors' forms of talk appear to be dependent therefore on both the patient's resistance to the treatment being proposed and on the doctor's conviction that the treatment being proposed is the best. Cordella (in press) suggests that doctors use different discourse strategies in response to a patient's reluctance to follow a proposed treatment, ranging from the brusque exercise of power to the use of *simpatía* as a buffer between the doctor's issuing of instructions and the patient's reception of those instructions. As noted above, no single approach can be stated categorically to foster greater compliance, even though patients in the Semi-structured inverviews expressed a strong dislike of doctors who were overtly superior and unrelaxed.

The concept of *simpatía* is presented here following Triandis et al. (1984) and the later work of Erzinger (1989, 1991). *Simpatía* was defined in Chapter 2 (pp. 18–20) as a particular quality of interaction among Spanish speakers that works to avoid inter-personal conflict in favour of a friendly and relaxed exchange. I am interested in the ways that *simpatía* manifested itself in the medical discourse that is the focus of this research among Chilean-Spanish speakers, and in particular to determine when *simpatía* functions as a friendly mask to hide persuasion and power, and when it appears to wear a *genuine* costume of friendliness in the conversation.

In Examples 43–47 we saw Dr. Ana encouraging her patient Carmen to attend psychotherapy sessions for her depression. A *marker of conditional inevitability* (*sería bueno*, "it would be good") at line 102, repeated at line 114 with an intensifying adverb of manner (*sería bien bueno*, "it would be very good"), show Dr. Ana using *simpatía* to influence her patient's decision. The patient has a number of misgivings about the treatment, and *simpatía* can be seen to avoid an open conflict, which could jeopardize the "working consensus" (Goffman 1959:21). The *marker of conditional inevitability* helps to create an atmosphere of friendliness in which the imposition (Brown & Levinson 1987) put on the patient is less explicit than in those cases where the *marker of inevitability* is used. In contrast, Example 48 showed Dr. Carlos delivering selective information and using intimidating discourse strategies in the absence of *simpatía*, particularly his conditional clause in line 146, *Si no se opera debe aceptar un poco esas limitaciones* ("If you don't have the operation you'll have to accept limitations").

Dr. Ana also displays *simpatía* in Example 41 when she suggests that Carmen attend *(El) Club de Tango o Centro de Madre lo que sea* ("(The) Tango Club or Mothers' Centre, whatever it may be") in line 228. Dr. Ana uses her *Educator voice* to persuade Carmen that the best way to deal with loneliness is to join a social group. We noted in Chapter 5 that the *Educator voice* in this episode reinforced the doctor's superior status and the expectations placed on women like Carmen in Chilean society. Nonetheless, *simpatía* is shown in the "disrupting" of a medical discourse by practical suggestions that have taken the patient's situation into account. (Mothers' Centres are usually formed by a group of women who get together regularly to share their experiences and make arts and crafts to raise money in the community. The Tango Club is a place where Carmen might meet a partner.) Both recommendations deconstruct a gender identity in a social setting (Holmes 1987, 1990, 1992, 1997; Pauwels 1987; Todd & Fisher 1988; West & Zimmerman 1991; Winter 1992; Winter & Wigglesworth 1993; Wodak 1997) by highlighting those social activities where a female of Carmen's age would be welcomed.

Although *simpatía* is a recurrent feature of Dr. Ana's consultation with Carmen, this does not mean that she fails to exercise her legitimate authority. We saw in her concluding remarks in Example 47 an assertion of her wishes in the *Doctor voice*, emphasized by specific usage of the first-person pronoun *yo* in line 119. Although they used very different discourse strategies, both Dr. Carlos and Dr. Ana made their wishes clear to the patient, and in so doing exercised their power and knowledge in the exchange.

9.4 Affiliative discourse and *simpatía*

Affiliative discourse was found in all three doctors' *voices* – *Doctor, Educator* and *Fellow Human*, but, as has been highlighted in this study, the latter presented many more discourse forms that expressed affiliation than the other two. Affiliative discourse strategies create empathy with the patient and promote a co-operative communication in which *simpatía* plays a central role. *Simpatía* can be seen as operating to make the interaction less symmetrical through the doctor's use of discourse forms that focus on building up a friendly relationship.

In the *Doctor voice* affiliation was achieved by doctors asking questions that were patient-oriented (as opposed to purely condition-oriented) and that centred on the impact the health condition was having on the patient's activities (see Example 7). In the *Fellow Human voice*, doctors showed affiliation by asking questions about the patient's lifeworld, such as work and family commitments, obligations and responsibilities. It is possible of course that doctors may use this type of questioning to gain a better understanding of the patient's health problem, recognizing that there may be a connection between a presenting physical illness and underlying emotional issues. Some psychological/psychiatric studies give support to the idea that illnesses are related to a person's environment in the broader sense (Stoudemire 1990). Nonetheless, it was clear from the data that asking these types of questions helped to create a more personal and caring interaction.

It is also worth stressing that it is not just the asking of the question itself that shows *simpatía*, but rather that *simpatía* develops around such keenly felt topics as divorce, funerals, difficulty with teenagers' behaviour, sibling relationships, money problems and work-related issues. There is the inherent risk in this that physicians may be drawn into conversations that fall outside their expertise, such as those that require the specialized knowledge of psychiatrists or social workers. In these instances, doctors must recognize their own limitations and refer the patient to a more appropriate treatment, as did Dr. Ana when she encouraged Carmen to attend psychotherapy for her depression. Another potential problem of engaging with the patient's lifeworld was made clear in Examples 49–51 when Olga told Dr. Carlos that *con algunas personas que han tenido este problema no te opere– que es horrible y fuera de eso al final uno queda igual* ("some people who've had the same problem (have said to me) don't have the operation, for it's horrible and, besides, it made no difference in the end"). Here Dr. Carlos's ideological convictions came into conflict with Carmen's reconting of her experiences, and his stronger need to express his views than to allow Carmen to continue as the main protagonist of her story resulted in an absence of *simpatía*.

In the *Educator voice* affiliation and *simpatía* were also present in some of the educative episodes as everyday language and colloquialisms that avoided arcane medical terminology (Examples 29 and 31) and helped the patient's learning process (Daly & Hulka 1975). As Goffman points out (1981), everyday talk is also less "restrained" than institutional dialogue and thus allows *simpatía* to be more readily expressed. In addition, the use of metaphors such as *sin gusto a nada* ("nothing was showing"/"in this case it was unclear"; literally, "without any taste") in Example 36, and *todavía no pasan balas por ahí* ("it [the patient's heart] is still bullet-proof") (Example 16), is an example of what Prieto-Castillo (1999) refers to as *el juego de la palabra* ("the playing with words") that occurs when informal speech is used. *Simpatía* can therefore function in the medically oriented discourse of *Doctor* and *Educator voices* as a parenthetical assortment of colloquialisms, metaphors and word-play.

So far we have looked at ways in which education is achieved in the consultation and observed the interconnection that appears to be present between education and the exercise of power. The selection of information given to the patient and the discourse developed in the process of communicating it can impose different degrees of power over the patient. The use of *simpatía* in medical discourse, then, seems to have two distinct functions: (a) the exercise of power is accomplished by using persuasive discourse forms, and (b) affiliation between doctor and patient is fostered in a friendly exchange, which encourages the patient's participation. This point is developed below.

The *Fellow Human voice* expresses a holistic approach to the patient's health, incorporating in the consultation both the socio-relational and the biomedical approaches to medicine. This *voice* favours communication where the patient can be heard, understood and can build up a relationship of trust with the doctor. *Simpatía* is mostly manifested in this *voice*. The absence of the *Fellow Human voice* is likely to produce discourse that shows a disregard for the individual who is after medical help by placing all the focus on the body part to be repaired. However, in this study the *Fellow Human voice* was used extensively and through it people were treated as both persons and patients whose illness and individual identity were all taken into consideration.

Previous studies of discourse analysis have interpreted "taking the floor" as a sign of the exercise of power over others. In the case of doctor–patient communication, interruptions have been understood as an attempt to (re)gain power in the medical interview. If taking the floor is a manifestation of assuming control over the conversation as well as over the other participant, situations in which doctors ask their patients to take the floor in order to elaborate and expand on their own stories can be recognized as an alternative or complement to their own exercise of power. The simple use of CMs (*ya, Mm/Uhm, Mm/Uhm ya*) in the data, produced in a low tone between patients' contributions, was indicative of doctors' willingness to hear their patients in an (apparently) unrushed consultation. CMs proved to be important in encouraging patients to talk about themselves while concomitantly showing them that they were being considered as both a person and a patient. Although in the majority of the consultations CMs called for patients' elaboration of their discourse, there were 3/261 examples where the patient was not willing to contribute further and the floor was given back to the doctor. Patients' inclusion of stories that sometimes appeared to be unrelated to their current health condition showed that medical discourse need not be only health-problem oriented but could permit the display of other discourses as well. One example of this was shown in the use of *joint production units* where both participants co-operated to construct a discourse together (Example 55). Following Ferrara (1992:208):

> The sentence itself can be viewed by interlocutors as a discourse unit under construction, because some speakers seize the opportunity to collaboratively shape discourse semantically and syntactically, one clause or phrase at a time, in the joint achievement of a sentence.

Doctors' co-operation to complete patients' discourse (Davis 1988; Todd & Fisher 1993) and finish their sentences is not interpreted as a paternalistic form, since no attempt is made to regain the floor or to impose a particular topic of conversation on the patient. Whereas *utterance extension* was represented in 68% of the joint production units found in the study, both *predictable utterance completion* and *helpful utterance completion* were less represented, with 16% each. The occurrence of these "collaborative" discourse markers, following Sacks's (1965–1971) term – regardless of their frequencies – appears to indicate that the doctors were not just helping to produce the discourse but in so doing they were creating a rapport from where the interaction could be developed. Ferrara, however, observed that there is a correlation between a long-standing relation and building of rapport and the frequency with which joint productions are used in the discourse (1992:213). Doctors' contributions in joint production units helped to make the discourse flow smoothly as if a conversation was being developed between people who knew each other relatively well. This supports Schegloff's views that "one person knows what the other person has in mind by saying it for him[/her] ... [s/he is] completing his[/her] sentence" (1984:42). Similarly, Marshall (1988) observed that co-operation in doctor and patient discourse resulted in the use of "duetting" and the building up of sentences. This point is also shared by Ochs et al. who, after observing the storytelling developed at a family dinner table, indicated that the familiarity with one another's narrative event, shared background knowledge as well as family bonds of trust, constituted fundamental elements that prompted individuals to participate in the joint construction of their stories. In their study the familiarity of participants elicited the joint construction, deconstruction and reconstruction of everyday activities. They argue that "more distant personal and professional relationships may very well inhibit the development of these skills" (Ochs et al. 1992: 67). In my study doctors indeed contributed to patients' discourse. My intention is not to equate joint production fully with the complex storytelling shown in Ochs et al.'s set of data, since my data do not show the same pattern. Nevertheless the joint productions that occur in this study represent a collaborative cognitive and socio-linguistic form that shows similarities of affiliation with the family discussions. Why joint productions appear in discourse as apparently far removed from family conversation as the medical interview is therefore of interest.

The use of joint production units may be interpreted as a precursor of the building up of trust between participants; it is a discourse strategy that is most likely found in informal or family get-togethers (Polanyi 1989; Shiffrin 1984; Tannen 1983, 1984). This also relates to Carmichael's findings that the presence of reciprocal family topics between doctors and patients is a sign of trust – "exposing one's unprotected part in a family relationship is not submission but evidence of trust" (1976: 562). If doctors avoid collaborative production of the discourse with their patients, this could be interpreted as a sign of distancing behaviour. It would be most in evidence if doctors did not contribute *helpful utterance completions*, as their silence could be interpreted as a reproach in response to the patient's forgetfulness for not being able to recall a word and thus needing the doctor to co-operate in the completion of the idea.

This study also indicates that the functions *Creating empathy* and *Showing special attentiveness* are used to create the same pleasant atmosphere that is found in friendly and familiar interactions. Patients feel that they are being heard and understood, and doctors can interact with the patient in a less asymmetrical manner by co-operating in the discourse. Following Erzinger, "attentive forms" represent a pivotal element in the elaboration of the patient's story and the key to success in the interaction:

> The most essential component of the doctor's conversational manner in medical encounters with Spanish-speaking patients is assuming an attitude of respectful listener. Where the patient is unable to expand upon her concerns, the doctor's careful paraphrasing and use of the patient's own words encourage elaboration. The patient's perception of the doctor's understanding, the key to successful interaction, depends upon how the patient is able to describe her concerns. (1988: 195)

This study suggests that the interaction is likely to be successful when both doctor and patient work together in the consultation to create a platform where the channel of communication is open to understand each other. The following section develops this point.

9.5 One consultation, two participants: An interactional work

The realization of the medical exchange is a twofold activity where both participants have the chance to modulate their speech within the communicative constraints of institutional talk. The interaction of participants and the *voices* used in their exchange appear to indicate a dichotomous system of operation where patients are both constrained and encouraged to participate in the medical discourse, and may exercise their individual discretion to act or otherwise. In this study patients had the chance to intervene and influence the course of an action (Giddens 1976), as well as show alignment to the expectations of the medical institution asked of them.

The participation of individuals is conditioned by and mainly constrained to the central aim of the medical consultation: that of getting information about the patient's health, making an assessment of his/her illness, and (if necessary) prescribing treatment. This explains the recurrent use of the *Doctor voice* and the number of questions addressed to the patient, whose answers are generally a function of the type of question asked. This implies that it is important for doctors to ask the "right" kinds of questions; that is, those which have the potential to provide the most relevant information that forms an integral part of building up the patient's medical history. Similarly, when patients perform the *voice* of *Initiator* they indicate their commitment to the medical institution and to their interest in understanding their health situation. As shown in Chapters 7 and 8, doctors responded to these questions by providing answers in the *Educator voice* and fulfilled their roles as experts of medical information.

Doctors and patients also show their mutual work through patients' compliance to the medical recommendations that may result in an improvement in their health condition. The importance of the *Educator voice* to achieve this end appears to be paramount when the literature of patient satisfaction and of compliance is taken into account.

The *Fellow Human voice* and the stories that develop within *Health-related storytelling* and *Social Communicator* present an interesting scenario of co-operation where the story that has been developed is the result of both participants' contribution. The doctor's use of discourse features that prompt the elaboration of the patient's discourse and the patient's development of the stories in response to the doctor's encouragement, represent the dual work that is taking place. As observed by Davis, "stories are not told, monologue-fashion to brick walls, but are collaborative achievements" (1988: 150). Following Goffman:

> Over the course of the interaction the roles of speaker and hearer will be interchanged in support of a statement-reply format, the acknowledged current-speaking right – the floor – passing back and forth. (1981: 129)

The collaboration I have been referring to so far is the product of an activity of communication that is influenced by both the *voices* participants use in an episode and the shift that may occur in subsequent episodes, which might have an impact on the recipient's use of *voices.*

In the participation framework of the medical consultation the shift of footing accords with both the interaction of participants, current practices in medicine and the institution in which the exchange takes place. The prevalent use of the *Doctor voice* in the history-taking and patients' response to it through the use of *voices* of *Health-related storytelling* and of *Competence*, account for the alignment that both participants have with respect to the medical exchange and to the restraints put on the relevant medical discourse to be developed. Doctors' shift to the *Educator voice* represents, in this study, their stance in the medical institution, by aligning themselves to the principles of a teaching hospital that trains doctors and patients (see Section 3.5). The use of *Doctor* or *Educator voice* is a response to the *voice* of *Initiator* by which the patients themselves align to their condition of unhealthy individuals and introduce a medical topic to be further developed. On the other hand, the *voice* of *Health-related storytelling* usually appears in the discourse after the *Doctor voice* has been introduced. The development of the *voice* of *Health-related storytelling* is associated with both the patient's interest in staying in that *voice* – regardless (in some instances) of the *voice* of the doctor, whether the *Fellow Human voice* that prompts the patient to continue, or a shift to the *Doctor voice* in order to resume questioning.

Whereas on the one hand patients responded to the medical *voices* enacted by doctors, on the other they diverged from them by introducing the *Social Communicator* and the *Initiator voices* without explicit openings or invitations in the talk. Those instances where the patients did not respond to the medical *voices* and performed as *Social Communicators* instead, showed that patients could control the topic they wanted to be developed. Indeed, patients' performance revealed a dual-dynamic as well as an individual system of operation. Their discourse was not always confined to their role as patients. On the contrary, they showed a mobility of action in the medical exchange, thus portraying both the image of the unhealthy individual in the use of stories revolving around their health, as well as the image of a fellow human being through stories related to social contexts. This produced a consultation where the interaction of both the bio-medical and socio-relational frames were part of the discourse. Similarly, in Coupland et al.'s study on consultation openings, it was observed that patients could conform to the medical frame or diverge from it:

> Socio-relational talk is initially normative, and patients as well as doctors play significant parts in negotiating how and when they should move into medically framed talk. Indeed, there are instances when it is patients rather than doctors who first act to move their talk into medical disclosure and diagnosis, and instances when doctors persist with a socio-relational frame when they have clear opportunities to move into medical talk. (1994: 119)

Whereas doctors appeared to present a clear pattern of behaviour in their use of *voices*, this was not always the case for patients (see Chapter 9). The lack of a distinct pattern of usage in patients' *voices* and the shift from one *voice* to another may be interpreted following Martinic, who claims that although the medical consultation is conditioned by the institutional talk, the production of the discourse is dependent on the interaction that is created at the local level of the consultation:

> *En efecto, la conversación, pese a situarse en un marco institucional, tiene una contingencia que es propia de la situación local creada y ratificada por los interlocutores en el momento de la entrevista y de la consulta.* (1996: 16)

> In fact the conversation, although it occurs within an institutional framework, has its own contingency that is unique to the local situation that is created and maintained by the interlocutors at the time of the interview and consultation.

It is possible to suggest that the presence of a non-recurrent pattern of patients' behaviour affords an opportunity for participants to create an interaction that responds to both patients' and doctors' needs. Conversely, the strictly institutional and medically oriented perspective gives privilege to the voice of medicine, i.e. *Doctor* and *Educator voices*. Thus, the local interaction created within the institutional medical exchange operates at a dynamic level that is both institutional and personal. Patients in this process may have the chance to receive individually tailored care throughout the development of the interaction. The practice of patients of not following a constant pattern of behaviour appears to be common and accepted by doctors, otherwise doctors, in their authority, would show greater resistance to this interactional discourse. According to Fairclough, this demeanour represents a:

> Common sense [that] gives us not only meaning systems, but also what we might call the "interactional routines" associated with particular discourse types – the conventional ways in which participants interact with each other ... It's generally only when things go wrong that they draw themselves to our attention. (1989:98)

Patients' non-recurrent pattern of behaviour appears to be central to the personalized consultation they may receive.

In relation to patients' gender and its effect on doctors' consultative style, it was shown in the data that doctors' personal communicative style tended to be more of a determining factor than whether the patient was male or female. This was the case, for example, when Dr. Carlos was recorded as using *QSI ones* with higher frequency than the other doctors, regardless of the gender of his patient (see Table 9). Similarly, it was found that although on the surface it appeared that male doctors tended to *facilitate the telling of patients' stories* more often with female patients, further analysis revealed that use of this discourse strategy was bound to the individual nature of particular consultations rather than to gender alone. This may suggest that participants' gender may not necessarily be accountable *per se* for the high production of a specific strategy but that the idiosyncratic use of conversational features by one of the participants may contribute to shaping part or all of the consultation.

The data shows that there are some instances where participants' gender and the nature of the interaction *may* be playing a role in the selection of discourse strategies that doctors use in the consultation. When reporting medical information, both female and male doctors scored a higher number of episodes when interacting with patients of the opposite sex, particularly female doctors with male patients. A possible explanation might be that female doctors are aware that men visit the medical centre less frequently than women, and so need more information condensed into a single consultation, while male doctors are responding to questions initiated by women (see the *Initiator voice*).

The interpretation of participants' preferential discourse strategies is given with caution due to the small number of consultations involved in this study and the differential medical experiences that the two female doctors had compared with their male colleagues. Nevertheless, as I have stated elsewhere, "The results offer a 'discursive behavioral tendency' of the group under investigation, but may also constitute part of the whole spectrum of discourse possibilities in the medical discourse" (Cordella in press).

In what follows I will expand on compliance and its effects on patients' competence.

9.6 Competence in the medical setting

Throughout this study I have shown how doctors and patients interact in the medical exchange, and how participants bring a set of *voices* to the consultation that frame the medical event and provide the opportunity for the emergence of the social context of patients' lives. My interest in this section is to expand on the medical competence that patients can attain in the exchange and the benefit that this could bring to both participants. The performance of the *voice* of *Competence* reveals that patients are familiar with their health condition and understand what they should do to improve their health status. Patients also show alignment to the medical recommendations and in so doing they show adult competence of looking after themselves. In contrast, the *voice* of *Initiator* represents an instance where the patient asks for knowledge to be imparted from their less powerful subject position of lacking knowledge in medical matters (Labov & Fanshel 1977). It is precisely this differential knowledge position that participants occupy that promotes the asymmetrical relationship of the interaction. Although asymmetry is more apparent in the *voice* of *Initiator*, this voice is also *fundamental* in the process of education and in making patients knowledgeable about their health condition. I understand the acquisition of competence as a process where the patient goes from powerless – the *voice* of *Initiator* – to powerful – the *voice* of *Competence* – after a series of medical consultations. The acquired medical knowledge can be used by the patients to better understand their own health problem, to better describe their medical concern to the doctor, to better care for themselves and to better communicate, whereby the asymmetry between participants will be diminished. In fact Barton highlights that it is lack of competence that creates a disruptive and asymmetrical discourse: "more specifically, it is in this interactional situation that asymmetrical communication may emerge" (2000: 271). Thus competence when welcomed and nurtured by doctors is likely to improve both patient's knowledge and communication between doctor and patient. This is consistent with Ainsworth-Vaughn's study, in which she found that cancer patients and their doctors benefited from a co-operative interaction:

> The physicians I studied often cooperated with patients' claims to power. Physicians can cooperate without compromising their own selves. Patients'

> appropriate efforts to take control of illness translate directly into better treatment and reduced demands on overburdened physicians. (1998: 190)

There is another benefit to be considered. Barton (2000: 265) in her study found that the length of the referral sequence was shorter and more efficient in those consultations where patients had experience and expertise in their medical problem. Consequently, patient competence not only encourages a better use of the doctor's time, but also makes available more time to provide further education to the patient and respond to any additional needs.

Following Goffman (1959), the *Initiator* could be said to represent patients' social mobility not in terms of status but rather in terms of knowledge. Patients' interest in knowing about their health status and becoming competent is not due (at least there is no evidence in my study) to a desire to get closer to some "sacred" place (Goffman 1959: 45), but simply to have more control over their own bodies and to make their own informed decision about the treatment to be undertaken.

In contrast, doctors' refusal or lack of willingness to educate patients, their exercise of territorial power that controls the discourse to dismiss patients' opinions when they are medically framed, and the provision of selective information on the treatment to be prescribed, lead to a situation in which the patient remains uninformed and uneducated about his/her condition, and is likely to have less chance of being compliant than those patients who participate in a more informative medical consultation (Daly & Hulka 1975).

The resistance to seeing doctors as educators could also be interpreted as a deliberate mystification of medical knowledge. Goffman (1959) recalls the Ponsonby's advice to the King of Norway in his campaign to gain more popularity among people:

> He intended, he said, to go as much as possible among the people and thought it would be popular if, instead of going in a motor car, he and Queen Maud were to use tramways. I told him frankly that I thought this would be a great mistake as familiarity bred contempt ... Every man liked to think what he would do, if he was a King. *People invested the Monarch with every conceivable virtue and talent.* They were bound therefore to be disappointed if they saw him going about like an ordinary man in the street. (my emphasis, 1959: 75)

This text serves as a useful metaphor to illustrate the idea that if doctors keep aloof from patients (and do not involve themselves in patients' education, for example), this may reinforce the impression that doctors possess a knowledge that is magnified to such a proportion that it lies completely out of reach of the average person. Although mystification can be a factor in doctors' behaviour, patients in my study had the chance to introduce questions to the discourse and in this *helpless temporary stage* were nonetheless able to shape their competence about their health in a dynamic way (Barton 2000; Giddens 1979, 1987; Maynard 1992; Ten Have 1991).

Female and male patients showed a relatively similar frequency in their *voice* of *Competence* (51.5% for females and 48.5% for males, see Table 26). Nevertheless, a more detailed analysis reveals that female patients, in contrast to males, contested and negotiated with their doctors the treatment to be undertaken.

The *voice* of *Initiator* presents a pattern that favours female patients' participation. Women asked many more questions (63.2%) than males (36.8%) (Table 26). Those patients who initiated questions received a relevant medical response that augmented their medical knowledge and which could later be used to negotiate with the doctor the course of action to be taken. If my interpretation is correct, then the female patients in this study will acquire a better understanding of their health in the long term and ultimately will have the chance to negotiate health issues (e.g. the best treatment) with their doctors. Unfortunately I cannot prove this conclusively in this study but it is tempting to propose some possible explanations that may account for this gender-related behaviour.

Anthropological medicine notes that one of the major female roles in most Western and non-Western societies is to look after the health of the family. Helman describes how the family constitutes the source of initial health practices during the diagnosis and treatment of a disease:

> The main arena of health care is the *family*; here most ill-health is recognized and then treated. It is the real site of primary health care in any society. In the family, as Chrisman [1977] points out, the main providers of health care are *women*, usually mothers or grandmothers, who diagnose most illnesses and treat them with the materials at hand. It has been estimated that about 70–90 per cent of health care takes place within this sector, in both Western and non-Western societies. (Helman's emphasis, 1994:65)

The knowledge that women acquire is passed from generation to generation to provide health care to their own family. Concomitantly, female patients pay higher number of visits to a medical centre than males (Helman 1994). In the outpatient Clinic of PUC for example, female patients visited the centre three times more frequently than males, making them more familiar with the context-situation of the interaction and more articulate in their medical discourse. Hein and Wodak found that "It turned out that half of the women gave a complete account while two-third of the men only used a sentence or less" (1987:48). Female awareness of medical problems and family commitment might have been the result of the high use of the *voice* of *Initiator* among female patients.

9.7 A dynamic model of doctor–patient communication

The main findings of this work can be summarized in a general model of doctor–patient communication that I term *dynamic*. I wish to emphasize the dynamic nature of the model as it depicts a process in time that can be accelerated or slowed down according to the specific circumstances of the case under study. Figure 13 depicts the model in its essential features. It is clear from this work that the doctor possesses an initial basis of power conferred to him/her by his/her training as a physician. This technical power immediately establishes an asymmetry between doctor and patient, illustrated by the difference in the size of the boxes enclosing doctor and patient. Through the *Educator voice*, however, doctors may be able to increase the medical knowledge of their patients, thus producing competent patients who will be able to express themselves through the *voice* of *Competence*. Clearly, the *voice* of *Competence* confers a relative increase of power to the patient, as illustrated by the hatched line enlarging the patient's box. A competent patient is then capable of contesting the doctor's power, to which the doctor may respond by simply ignoring the patient or by entering into a negotiation with the patient that produces a more accurate feedback between interactants. Such feedback should be intended as a constructive one leading to a better understanding of the patient's health condition. This process, repeated over time, can set the stage for a positive feedback loop, leading to increasingly better informed doctors and increasingly more competent patients, which can improve the quality of the treatment, the rate of compliance and therefore the success of the healing process. Competence and negotiation should therefore lead to a more personal tailoring of the treatment.

Doctors can use two other *voices* in their interactions with patients. The *Fellow Human voice* establishes a co-operative communication between doctor and patient that unfolds in a process characterized by *simpatía*, i.e. expressions of friendliness and conflict-avoidance. To this *voice*, the patient usually responds with the use of *Health-related storytelling*, the *Social Communicator* and the *Initiator voices*. The *Doctor voice* is used in order to gather information, assess test results and assess the patient's compliance. The patient may interact

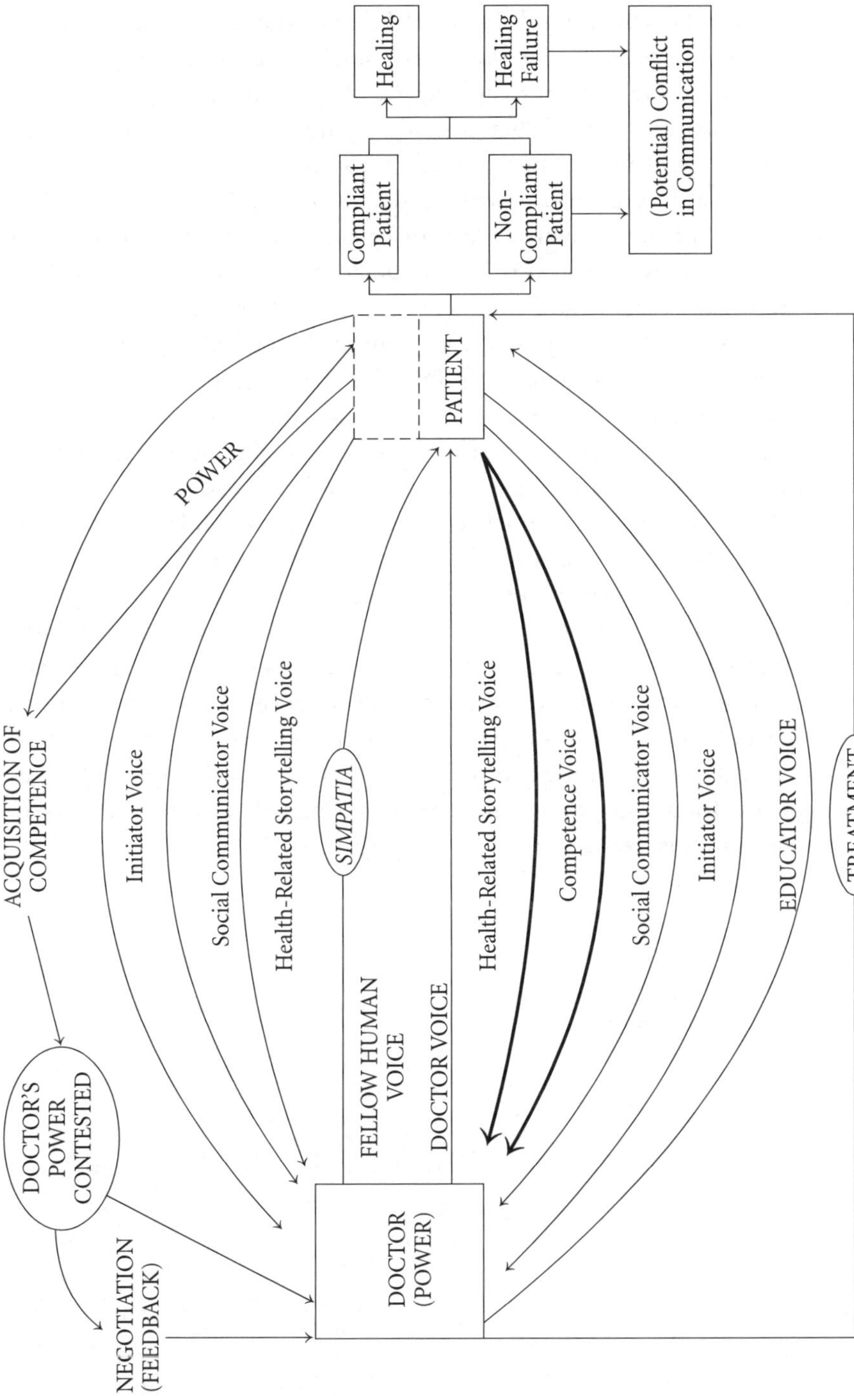
Healing
Healing Failure
Compliant Patient
Non-Compliant Patient
(Potential) Conflict in Communication
PATIENT
POWER
ACQUISITION OF COMPETENCE
Initiator Voice
Social Communicator Voice
Health-Related Storytelling Voice
SIMPATIA
Health-Related Storytelling Voice
Competence Voice
Social Communicator Voice
Initiator Voice
EDUCATOR VOICE
TREATMENT
DOCTOR'S POWER CONTESTED
FELLOW HUMAN VOICE
DOCTOR VOICE
NEGOTIATION (FEEDBACK)
DOCTOR (POWER)

with the *Doctor voice* by using the *voice* of *Initiator* (i.e. to ask medical questions), the *voice* of *Social Communicator* (i.e. to tell issues concerning personal life) and, above all, the *voices of Health-related storytelling* (i.e. the description, more or less elaborated, of his/her condition) and *Competence* (i.e. to show understanding of and alignment to medical recommendations).

Communication breakdown between doctor and patient is also possible. Such possibility of breakdown is likely to be diffused, that is, it may occur anywhere in the network of *voices* linking doctor and patient. In my study, I did not record any instances of complete communication breakdown such as would lead to the end of doctor–patient communication during the consultation. Tensions in doctor–patient communication may arise, however, as a result of the patient's lack of compliance with the prescribed treatment (doctor's perspective) or the patient's failure to achieve healing in spite of complying with the treatment recommended by the doctor (patient's perspective).

This study has shown that medical consultations in a Chilean setting display a participation framework in which both doctor and patient can author distinctive *voices*. The realization of those *voices* in the interaction projects both participants' alignments to the medical institution as well as individual stances reflecting their socio-cognitive understanding of the event. The interaction between *voices* that emerges during the consultation appears to be pivotal in the development of doctor–patient communication. In the final chapter I derive some general conclusions from this research and set the stage for a general analytical framework that may serve as a point of reference for further investigations in this field.

Note

1. See www.puc.cl → Admisión.

Chapter 10

Concluding remarks

The aim of this study was to understand how communication between doctor and patient developed during medical consultations in an institutional setting in Chile. In this conclusion I highlight the implications of the findings by stressing the dynamic and productive communication that can be achieved when both participants know how to contribute more effectively to the discourse.

The interaction between doctors' and patients' *voices* in the medical discourse reveals participants' social identity and institutional alignments that can set them apart – by increasing the asymmetry in the event – or, conversely, can make them come closer (communicatively) in the discourse – by decreasing the asymmetry in the event.

The representation of the *Educator voice* is one example where the initial asymmetry is seen as just a starting point that marks the beginning of a process, which could achieve a more symmetrical communication over time. This knowledge-acquisition process would be fuelled by the relevant health information patients receive in their visits. As a consequence of the above learning process, the patient may develop competence which, if uncontested, can have remarkable implications in terms of negotiation of treatment and, ultimately, on the patient's compliance and (hopefully) healing. Nevertheless the *Educator voice* cannot by itself satisfy the overall needs of the consultation. This requires both the *Doctor voice* and the *Fellow Human voice*, that provide the essential tools for a holistic understanding of patients' health, throughout the discourse types that investigate the patient's health condition and the discourse strategies that facilitate the recounting of patients' own stories.

In this process of seeking information (*Doctor voice*), educating (*Educator voice*) and using strategies to facilitate patients' talk (*Fellow Human voice*), patients show alignment to the medical institution (the *voices* of *Health-related storytelling* and *Competence*), interest in further understanding their health condition (the *voice* of *Initiator*) and interest in sharing their personal stories (the *voice* of *Social communicator*). As a consequence, the communication develops as a *dynamic system* where some *voices* restrict the participation of patients (increasing the asymmetry in the event), while other facilitate their contribution (decreasing the asymmetry in the event). This dynamic system operates within a range of different degrees of asymmetry that vary from the blunt exercise of power, which augments asymmetry, to the subtle expressions of power that moderate and diminish the asymmetry. This dynamic development of the consultation creates the participation framework that doctors and patients move in, and allows both power and *simpatía* to be represented during the consultation.

The communication between doctor and patient appears to reflect Chilean socio-cultural values and ideologies that are reproduced at the micro level of the interaction. Thus, doctors show their authority by using persuasive discourse strategies to reinforce their opinions on what patients' medical treatment should be, as well as to exert influence on patients' cognitive perception of society. In other words doctors, in their performance as health professionals, express personal opinions that are framed in the medical context, and so their own ideologies permeate the discourse. Similarly, patients also show their alignment to the socio-cultural group where they belong by developing the voice of the *Social Communicator* and incorporating in their discourse themes that reflect their value system. The *voice* of *Initiator* could also be interpreted in terms of social mobility, since the patients by initiating the talk and taking the floor author a voice of control in the event, but most importantly the *voice* of *Initiator* shows that both doctors and patients can be *heard* in the consultation.

Following Wodak (1989), in order to bring changes to institutional practices there is a need to give a *diagnosis* of the participation framework of individuals and propose a *therapy* that will (hopefully) ameliorate the deficiencies of the institutional practice under investigation. The *Educator voice* appears to be fundamental to make patients more aware of their health condition and to give them more control over their treatment, nonetheless not every consultation provided educative episodes. This may suggest that there is a need to address health issues at different levels. First of all there is a need to train doctors in the *subtle art* of training patients to become more aware and knowledgeable about their own health. Special emphasis should be given to: how to better convey biological and medical knowledge, how to make patients aware of health issues associated with a varied spectrum of lifestyles, how to educate patients to seek proper professional advice on time, how to self-monitor the development of a disease state, how to interpret the severity of the symptoms being experienced.

Although public health campaigns on preventative medicine address most of the points illustrated above, it is in the medical consultation that the knowledge acquired through other means can be consolidated. To disconnect public awareness campaigns on health (i.e. quitting smoking, reducing fat intake) from the medical consultation may only augment the chances of having patients who ignore early signs of a disease. Secondly, the benefits of such a patient-empowering programme are likely to feedback onto the medical system by improving the quality of information doctors have at hand to establish their diagnosis and treatment. Moreover, the ability of patients to effectively and safely monitor their health condition, and to prevent disease states occurring in the first place, may relieve the health system from excessive pressure, thus making the possibly limited resources (especially in economically depressed regions) available preferably to those patients that really need them. This may be beneficial in terms of shortening queueing times at health care centres. Studies in discourse analysis, with a critical analysis approach, can be of great help in this process, as they may provide practical advice on improving the ability of patients to articulate their concerns and of doctors to improve their communication abilities.

Future studies should give special attention to research on the *Educator voice* in order to further understand the interaction that develops between doctor and patient when this *voice* is present in the consultation. In addition, future studies should also investigate diachronically the effect of patients' medical competence and its outcomes on the medical system and on the interaction developed with health professionals. If the efficient use of resources available to health systems is a social desideratum, then there is a need to better educate people to be more competent about medical issues.

Bibliography

Adler, S., S. McGraw, & J. McKinlay (1998). "Patient assertiveness in ethnically diverse older women with breast cancer: challenging stereotypes of the elderly". *Journal of Aging Studies, 12,* 331–350.

Ainsworth-Vaughn, N. (1994). "Negotiating genre and power: Questions in medical discourse". In B. L. Gunnarsson, P. Linell, & B. Nordstrom (Eds.), *Text and Talk in Professional Contexts* (pp. 149–166). Uppsala, Sweden: Association Suédoise de Linguistique Appliquée.

Ainsworth-Vaughn, N. (1998). *Claiming Power in Doctor–Patient Talk.* Oxford: Oxford University Press.

Andary, L., Y. Stolk, & S. Klimidis (2003). *Assessing Mental Health Across Cultures.* Bowen Hills, Qld: Australian Academic Press.

Aronsson, K., & B. Rundström (1989). "Cats, dogs, and sweets in the clinical negotation of reality: On politeness and coherence in pediatric discourse". *Language in Society, 18,* 483–504.

Atkinson, J. M. (1992). "Displaying neutrality: Formal aspects of informal court proceedings". In P. Drew & J. Heritage (Eds.), *Talk at Work: Interaction in Institutional Settings* (pp. 199–211). Cambridge: Cambridge University Press.

Atkinson, P. (1995). *Medical Talk and Medical Work: The Liturgy of the Clinic.* London: Sage Publications.

Austin, J. L. (1962). *How To Do Things With Words.* Oxford: Clarendon Press.

Bamberg, M. (1991). "Voices of curing and caring: The role of vagueness and ambiguity in informed consent discussions". *Family Systems Medicine, 9,* 329–342.

Barry, C. A., F. A. Stevenson, N. Britten, N. Barber, & C. P. Bradley (2001). "Giving voice to the lifeworld. More humane, more effective medical care? A qualitative study of doctor–patient communication in general practice". *Social Science and Medicine, 53,* 487–505.

Barton, E. L. (2000). "The interactional practice of referrals and accounts in medical discourse: expertise and compliance". *Discourse Studies, 2,* 259–281.

Beach, W. (2001). "Stability and ambiguity: Managing uncertain moments when updating news about Mom's cancer". *Text: An Interdisciplinary Journal for the Study of Discourse, 21,* 221–250.

Bensing, J. (1991). "Doctor–patient communication and the quality of care". *Social Science and Medicine, 32* (11), 1301–1310.

Bergmann, J. R. (1992). "Veiled morality: Notes on discretion in psychiatry". In P. Drew & J. Heritage (Eds.), *Talk at Work: Interaction in Institutional Settings* (pp. 137–162). Cambridge: Cambridge University Press.

Bissell, P., C. R. May, & P. R. Noyce (2004). "From compliance to concordance: Barriers to accomplishing a re-framed model of health care interactions". *Social Science and Medicine, 58* (4), 851–862.

Blanchard, C., M. Labrecque, & J. Ruckdeschel (1988). "Information decision-making preferences of hospitalized adult cancer patients". *Social Science Medicine, 27* (11), 1139–1145.

Blaxter, M. (1987). "Evidence on inequality in health from a national survey". *Lancet, 2*, 30–33.

Borges, S. (1986). "A feminist critique of scientific ideology". In S. Fisher & A. D. Todd (Eds.), *Discourse and Institutional Authority: Medicine, Education and Law* (pp. 26–48). Norwood, NJ: Ablex.

Brown, P., & S. Levinson (1987). *Politeness*. Cambridge: Cambridge University Press.

Buller, M. K., & D. B. Buller (1987). "Physicians' communication style and patient satisfaction". *Journal of Health Social Behaviour, 28*, 375–388.

Burgoon, M., T. Birk, & J. Hall (1991). "Compliance and satisfaction with physician–patient communication. An expectancy theory interpretation of gender differences". *Human Communication Research, 18*, 177–208.

Butt, J., & C. Benjamin (1988). *A New Grammar of Modern Spanish*. London: Edward Arnold.

Byrne, P., & B. Long (1976). *Doctors Talking to Patients*. London: HMSO.

Cameron, D. (1992). "'Respect, please!': Investigating race, power and language". In D. Cameron, E. Fraser, P. Harvey, M. B. H. Rampton, & K. Richardson (Eds.), *Researching Language Issues of Power Method* (pp. 113–138). London: Routledge.

Cameron, D. (2001). *Working with Spoken Discourse*. London: Sage Publications.

Carmichael, L. P. (1976). "The family in medicine, process or entity?" *Journal of Family Practice, 3*, 562–563.

Carranza, I. E. (1998). *Conversación y Deixis de Discurso*. Córdoba: Universidad Nacional de Córdoba.

Cassell, E., L. Skopek, & B. Fraser (1976). "A preliminary model for the examination of doctor–patient communication". *Language Science, 43*, 10–13.

Charles, C., A. Gafni, & T. Whelan (1997). "Shared decision-making in the medical encounter: What does it mean?". *Social Science and Medicine, 44*, 681–692.

Charon, R., M. G. Greene, & R. D. Adelman (1994). "Multidimensional interaction analysis. A collaborative approach to the study of medical discourse". *Social Science and Medicine, 39* (7), 955–965.

Chrisman, N. J. (1977). "The health seeking process: An approach to the natural history of illness". *Culture, Medicine and Psychiatry, 1*, 351–377.

Cicourel, A. V. (1975). "Discourse and text: Cognitive and linguistic processes in studies of social structure". *Versus Quaderni di Studi Semiotici, 12*, 33–84.

Cicourel, A. V. (1981). "Notes on the integration of micro and macro levels of analysis". In K. D. Knorr-Cetina & A. V. Cicourel (Eds.), *Advances in Social Theory and Methodology: Toward an Integration of Micro and Macro Sociologies* (pp. 51–80). Boston: Routledge and Kegan Paul.

Cicourel, A. V. (1995). "Medical speech events as resources for inferring differences in expert–novice diagnostic reasoning". In Uta M. Quasthoff (Ed.), *Aspects of Oral Communication* (pp. 364–387). Berlin and New York: Walter de Gruyter.

Cicourel, A. V. (1999). "The interaction of cognitive and cultural models in health care delivery". In S. Sarangi & C. Roberts (Eds.), *Talk, Work and Institutional Order. Discourse in Medical, Mediation and Management Settings* (pp. 183–224). Berlin: Mouton de Gruyter.

Coates, J. (1996). *Women Talk. Conversation Between Women Friends.* Oxford: Blackwell.

Coates, J. (Ed.). (1998). *Language and Gender. A Reader.* Oxford: Blackwell.

Cohen-Cole, S. A. (1991). *The Medical Interview: The Three-Function Approach.* St. Louis, Baltimore: Mosby Year Book.

Cohen-Cole, S. A. (1994). "The biopsychosocial model in medical practice". In A. Stoudemire (Ed.), *Human Behavior: An Introduction* (pp. 3–30). Philadelphia: J. B. Lippincott.

Cordella, M. (1990). "Apologizing in Chilean Spanish and Australian English: A cross-cultural perspective". *Australian Review of Applied Linguistics, Series S* (7), 66–92.

Cordella, M. (1991). "Spanish speakers apologizing in English: A cross-cultural pragmatics study". *Australian Review of Applied Linguistics, 14,* 115–138.

Cordella, M. (1992). "Travels, cultures and speech acts: A pragmatics study in apology". *The Ken Garrad Working Papers in Hispanic Studies* 2. Clayton, Vic.: Monash University.

Cordella, M. (1996). "Confrontational style in Spanish arguments: pragmatics outlook". *Language, Culture and Curriculum, 9,* 148–162.

Cordella, M. (1999). "Medical discourse in a Hispanic environment: Power and *simpatía* under investigation". *Australian Review of Applied Linguistics, 22* (2), 35–50.

Cordella, M. (2003). "En el corazón del debate: el análisis del discurso en la representación de las voces médicas". *Oralia. Análsis del discurso oral, 6,* 147–168.

Cordella, M. (in press). "'No, no I haven't been taking it doctor': Compliance, face threatening acts and politeness in medical consultations". In M. Placencia & C. García (Eds.), *Linguistic Politeness in the Spanish-Speaking World.* Mahwah, NJ: Lawrence Erlbaum Associates.

Cordella, M., & K. Forbes (1998). "Discourse control and leadership in conflict talk". *Onomázein: Revista de Lingüística, Filología y Traducción del Instituto de Letras de la Pontificia Universidad Católica de Chile, 3,* 45–61.

Cordella, M., H. Large, & V. Pardo (1995). "Complimenting behaviour in Australian English and Spanish speech". *Multilingua: Journal of Cross-Cultural and Interlanguage Communication, 14,* 235–252.

Corsaro, W. A. (1982). "Something old and something new: The importance of prior ethnography in the collection and analysis of audiovisual data". *Sociological Methods and Research, 2,* 145–166.

Coulthard, M., & M. Ashby (1975). "Talking with the doctor, 1". *Journal of Communication, 25,* 140–145.

Coulthard, M., & M. Ashby (1976). "A linguistic description of doctor–patient interviews". In M. Wadsworth & D. Robinson (Eds.), *Studies in Everyday Medical Life* (pp. 69–88). London: Martin Robertson.

Coupland, J., J. Robinson, & N. Coupland (1994). "Frame negotiation in doctor–elderly patient consultations". *Discourse and Society, 5*, 89–124.

Craib, I. (1992). *Anthony Giddens*. London: Routledge.

Daly, M., & B. Hulka (1975). "Talking with the doctor, 2". *Journal of Communication, 25* (30), 148–152.

Davis, K. (1988). *Power under the Microscope*. Dordrecht: Foris.

Dawson, M. T., S. Gifford, & R. Amezquita (2000). "¿Dónde hay doctor?: Folk and cosmopolitan medicine for sexual health among Chilean women living in Australia". *Culture, Health and Sexuality, 2*, 51–68.

Donovan, J. L., & D. R. Blake (1992). "Patient noncompliance–deviance or reasoned decision-making". *Social Science and Medicine, 34* (5), 507–513.

Dowsett, S. M., J. L. Saul, P. N. Butow, S. M. Dunn, M. J. Boyer, R. Findlow, & J. Dunsmore (2000). "Communication styles in the cancer consultation: preferences for a patient-centred approach". *Psycho-Oncology, 9*, 147–156.

Drew, P. (2001). "Spotlight on the patient". *Text: An Interdisciplinary Journal for the Study of Discourse, 21*, 261–268.

Drew, P., & A. Wootton (1988). "Introduction". In P. Drew & A. Wootton (Eds.), *Erving Goffman: Exploring the Interaction Order* (pp. 1–13). Cambridge: Polity Press.

Du Bois, J. (1991). "Transcription design principles for spoken discourse research". *Pragmatics, 1*, 71–106.

Engel, G. L. (1974). "The need for a new medical model: A challenge for biomedicine". *Science, 196* (12), 9–136.

Epstein, R. M., T. L. Campbell, S. A. Cohen-Cole, I. R. McWhinney, & G. Smilkstein (1993). "Perspectives on patient–doctor communication". *Journal of Family Practice, 37*, 377–388.

Erickson, F., & J. Shultz (1982). *The Counselor as Gatekeeper. Social Interaction in Interview*. New York: Academic Press.

Erzinger, S. (1989). "Consultas médicas: A Study of Communication between Spanish Speaking Patients and their Doctors". Unpublished doctoral dissertation, University of California at Berkeley.

Erzinger, S. (1991). "Communication between Spanish-speaking patients and their doctors in medical encounters". *Culture, Medicine and Psychiatry, 15*, 91–110.

Fairclough, N. (1985). "Critical and descriptive goals in discourse analysis". *Journal of Pragmatics, 9*, 739–763.

Fairclough, N. (1989). *Language and Power*. London: Longman.

Fairclough, N. (1992). *Discourse and Social Change*. Cambridge: Polity Press.

Fairclough, N. (1995). *Critical Analysis: The Critical Study of Language*. London: Longman.

Fairclough, N., & R. Wodak (1997). "Critical discourse analysis". In T. A. van Dijk (Ed.), *Discourse as Social Interaction* (pp. 258–284). London: Sage.

Falk, J. (1980). "The conversational duet". In B. R. Caron et al. (Eds.), *Proceedings of the Sixth Annual Meeting of the Berkeley Linguistics Society* (pp. 507–514). Berkeley: University of California.

Ferrara, K. (1992). "The interactive achievement of a sentence: Joint productions in therapeutic discourse". *Discourse Processes, 15*, 207–228.

Fisher, S. (1991). "A discourse of the social: Medical talk / power talk / oppositional talk?". *Discourse and Society, 2*, 157–182.

Fisher, S. (1993). "Doctor talk / patient talk: How treatment decisions are negotiated in doctor–patient communication". In A. D. Todd & S. Fisher (Eds.), *The Social Organization of Doctor–Patient Communication* (pp. 161–182). Norwood, NJ: Ablex.

Fisher, S. (1995). *Nursing Wounds: Nurse Practitioners, Doctors, Women Patients and the Negotiation of Meaning*. New Brunswick, NJ: Rutgers University Press.

Fisher, S., & S. Groce (1985). "Doctor–patient negotiation of cultural assumptions". *Sociology of Health and Illness, 7*, 342–374.

Fisher, S., & S. Groce (1990). "Accounting practices in medical interviews". *Language in Society, 19*, 225–250.

Fisher, S., & A. D. Todd (Eds.). (1983). *The Social Organization of Doctor–Patient Communication*. Washington, DC: Center for Applied Linguistics Press.

Fisher, S., & A. D. Todd (Eds.). (1986a). *Discourse and Institutional Authority: Medicine, Education, and Law*. Norwood, NJ: Ablex.

Fisher, S., & A. D. Todd (1986b). "Friendly persuasion: Negotiating decisions to use oral contraceptives". In S. Fisher & A. D. Todd (Eds.), *Discourse and Institutional Authority: Medicine, Education, and Law* (pp. 3–25). Norwood, NJ: Ablex.

Forbes, K., & M. Cordella (1999). "The role of gender in Chilean argumentative discourse". *International Review of Applied Linguistics in Language Teaching, 37*, 277–289.

Foucault, M. (1975). *The Birth of the Clinic: An Archeology of Medical Perception*. New York: Vintage Books.

Foucault, M. (1980). *Power/Knowledge: Selected Interviews and Other Writings 1972–1977*. London: Harvester Books.

Frankel, R. (1984). "Physicians and patients in social interaction: Medical encounters as a discourse process". *Discourse Processes, 7*, 103–224.

Frankel, R. (1990). "Talking in interviews: A dispreference for patient-initiated questions in physician–patient encounters". In G. Psathas (Ed.), *Everyday Language: Studies in Ethnomethodology* (pp. 231–262). New York: Irvington.

Gabbardalley, A. (1995). "Health communication and gender: A review and critique". *Health Communication, 7*, 35–54.

Gerber, K. (1986). "Compliance in the chronically ill: An introduction to the problem". In K. Gerber & A. Nehemkis (Eds.), *Compliance: The Dilemma of the Chronically Ill* (pp. 13–23). New York: Springer.

Giaconi, J. (1994). "El sistema de salud chileno". *Boletín Escuela de Medicina, Pontificia Universidad Católica de Chile, 23*, 6–9.

Giddens, A. (1976). *New Rules of Sociological Method. A Positive Critique of Interpretative Sociologies*. London: Hutchinson.

Giddens, A. (1977). *Studies in Social and Political Theory*. London: Hutchinson.

Giddens, A. (1979). *Central Problems in Social Theory*. London: MacMillan.

Giddens, A. (1981). *A Contemporary Critique of Historical Materialism*. London: MacMillan.

Giddens, A. (1984). *The Constitution of Society*. Cambridge: Polity Press.

Giddens, A. (1987). *Social Theory of Modern Sociology*. Stanford, CA: Stanford University Press.

Gill, V. T., T. Halkowski, & F. Roberts (2001). "Accomplishing a request without making one: A single case analysis of a primary care visit". *Text: An Interdisciplinary Journal for the Study of Discourse, 21*, 55–81.

Goffman, E. (1959). *The Presentation of Self in Everyday Life*. London: Penguin.

Goffman, E. (1963). *Behavior in Public Places. Notes on the Social Organization of Gatherings*. New York: Free Press.

Goffman, E. (1967). *Interactional Ritual Essays on Face-to-Face Behavior*. New York: Pantheon Books.

Goffman, E. (1971). *Relations in Public. Micro-Studies of the Public Order*. New York: Harper and Row.

Goffman, E. (1981). *Forms of Talk*. Philadelphia: University of Pennsylvania Press.

Goffman, E. (1983). "The interaction order". *American Sociological Review, 48*, 1–17.

Gopinath, B., K. Radhakrishnan, P. S. Sarma, D. Jayachandran, & A. Alexander (2000). "A questionnaire survey about doctor–patient communication: Compliance and locus of control among South Indian people with epilepsy". *Epilepsy Research, 39*, 73–82.

Grainger, K. (2002). "Politeness or impoliteness?: Verbal play on the hospital ward". *Working Papers on the Web*, Vol. 3 (*Linguistic Politeness and Context*) <www.shu.ac.uk/wpw/politeness/grainger.htm> (accessed April 2004)

Grice, H. P. (1971 (1957)). "Meaning". In D. D. Steinberg & L. A. Jakobovits (Eds.), *Semantics: An Interdisciplinary Reader in Philosophy, Linguistics and Psychology* (pp. 53–59). Cambridge: Cambridge University Press.

Grimshaw, A. (1981). *Language as Social Resource*. Stanford, CA: Stanford University Press.

Gruninger, U. J. (1995). "Patient education: An example of one-to-one communication". *Journal of Human Hypertension, 1*, 15–25.

Gumperz, J. (1971). *Language in Social Groups: Essays by John Gumperz*. Stanford, CA: Stanford University Press.

Gumperz, J. (1982a). *Discourse Strategies*. Cambridge: Cambridge University Press.

Gumperz, J. (Ed.). (1982b). *Language and Social Identity*. Cambridge: Cambridge University Press.

Gumperz, J. (1999). "On interactional sociolinguistic method". In S. Sarangi & C. Roberts (Eds.), *Talk, Work and Institutional Order. Discourse in Medical, Mediation and Management Settings* (pp. 453–471). Berlin: Mouton de Gruyter.

Gumperz, J., & D. Hymes (Eds.). (1972). *Directions in Sociolinguistics: The Ethnography of Communication*. New York, Chicago: Holt Rinehart and Winston.

Haakana, M. (2001). "Laughter as a patient's resource: Dealing with delicate aspects of medical interviews". *Text: An Interdisciplinary Journal for the Study of Discourse, 21*, 187–219.

Haberland, H., & J. L. Mey (1981). "Wording and warding: The pragmatics of therapeutical conversation". *Journal of Pragmatics, 5*, 103–111.

Hadlow, J., & M. Pitts (1991). "The understanding of common health terms by doctors, nurses and patients". *Social Science and Medicine, 32*, 193–196.

Hahn, R. A. (1995). *Sickness and Healing. An Anthropological Perspective*. Yale University Press.

Harres, A. (1996). "Tag Questions and Gender in Medical Consultations". Unpublished doctoral dissertation, Monash University.

Harres, A. (1998). "'But basically you're feeling well, are you?': Tag questions in medical consultations". *Health Communication, 10*, 111–123.

Heath, C. (1992). "The delivery and reception of diagnosis in the general-practice consultation". In P. Drew & J. Heritage (Eds.), *Talk at Work: Studies in Interactional Sociolinguistics 8* (pp. 235–267). Cambridge: Cambridge University Press.

Hein, N. R., & Wodak (1987). "Medical interviews in internal medicine. Some results of an empirical investigation". *Text: An Interdisciplinary Journal for the Study of Discourse, 7*, 37–66.

Helman, C. G. (1994). *Culture, Health and Illness: An Introduction for Health Professionals* (3rd ed.). Oxford: Butterworth-Heinemann.

Holmes, J. (1987). "Hedging, fencing and other conversational gambits: An analysis of gender differences in New Zealand speech". In A. Pauwels (Ed.), *Women and Language in Australian and New Zealand Society* (pp. 59–79). Sydney: Australian Professional Publications.

Holmes, J. (1990). "Hedges and boosters in women's and men's speech". *Language and Communication, 10*, 185–205.

Holmes, J. (1992). "Women's talk in public contexts". *Discourse and Society, 3*, 131–150.

Holmes, J. (1997). "Women, language and identity". *Journal of Sociolinguistics, 1*, 195–223.

Holmes, J., M. Stubbe, & B. Vine (1999). "Constructing professional identity: 'Doing power' in policy units". In S. Sarangi & C. Roberts (Eds.), *Talk, Work and Institutional Order. Discourse in Medical, Mediation and Management Settings* (pp. 351–386). Berlin and New York: Mouton de Gruyter.

Holquist, M. (1981). *The Dialogic Imagination: Four Essays by M. M. Bakhtin*. Austin: University of Texas Press.

Hymes, D. (1972). "On communicative competence". In J. B. Pride & J. Holmes (Eds.), *Sociolinguisics: Selected Readings* (pp. 269–293). Harmondsworth: Penguin.

Irish, J. T., & J. A. Hall (1995). "Interruptive patterns in medical visits: The effects of role, status and gender". *Social Science and Medicine, 41* (6), 873–881.

Jefferson, G. (1979). "A technique for inviting laughter and its subsequent acceptance declination". In G. Psathas (Ed.), *Everyday Language: Studies in Ethnomethodology* (pp. 79–96). New York: Irvington.

Jefferson, G. (1984). "On the organization of laughter in talk about trouble". In J. M. Atkinson & J. Heritage (Eds.), *Structure and Social Action* (pp. 346–369). Cambridge: Cambridge University Press.

Jefferson, G., H. Sacks, & E. Schegloff (1977). *Preliminary Notes on the Sequential Organization of Laughter*. Cambridge: Department of Linguistics, Cambridge University.

Jones, C. M. (2001). "Missing assessments: Lay and professional orientations in medical interviews". *Text: An Interdisciplinary Journal for the Study of Discourse, 21*, 113–150.

Jurafsky, D., E. Shriberg, B. Fox, & T. Curl (1998). "Lexical, prosodic, and syntactic cues for dialog acts". In *Proceedings of ACL/COLING-98 Workshop on Discourse Relations and Discourse Markers* (pp. 114–120). Montreal.

Kess, J. (1984). "Medical interviews and doctor–patient discourse. Review article". *Semiotica, 68*, 165–173.

Kleinman, A. (1980). *Patients and Healers in the Context of Culture: An Exploration of the Borderland between Anthropology, Medicine and Psychiatry*. Berkeley: University of California Press.

Kline, F., & F. Acosta (1980). "The misunderstood Spanish-speaking patient". *American Journal of Psychiatry, 137* (2), 1530–1533.

Korsch, B. M., E. K. Gozzi, & V. Francis (1968). "Gaps in doctor–patient communication: Doctor–patient interaction and patient satisfaction". *Pediatrics, 42*, 855–871.

Kreps, G. L. (1988). "Relational communication in health care". *Southern Communication Journal, 53*, 344–359.

Labov, W., & D. Fanshel (1977). *Therapeutic Discourse: Psychotherapy as Conversation*. New York: Academic Press.

Lacoste, M. (1981). "The old woman and the doctor: A contribution to the analysis of unequal linguistic exchange". *Journal of Pragmatics, 5*, 169–180.

Lebarère, J., J. P. Torres, P. François, M. Fourny, P. Argento, X. Gensburger, & P. Menthonnex (2003). "Patient compliance with medical advice by telephone". *The American Journal of Emergency Medicine, 21*, 288–292.

León, F. (2000). "The case of the Chilean health system 1983–2000". <www.who.int/trade/en/THpart3chap12.pdf> (accessed April 2004)

Levinson, S. (1983). *Pragmatics*. Cambridge: Cambridge University Press.

Levinson, S. (1988). "Putting linguistics on a proper footing: Explorations in Goffman's concept of participation". In P. Drew & A. Wootton (Eds.), *Erving Goffman: Exploring the Interaction Order* (pp. 161–227). Abingdon: Polity Press.

Lerner, G. (1991). "On the syntax of sentences-in-progress". *Language in Society, 20*, 441–458.

Lieberman, J. A. (1996). "Compliance issues in primary care". *Journal of Clinical Psychiatry, 57* (7), 76–85.

Littlewood, R. (1999). "Agency, opposition and resistance: a systemic approach to psychological illness in sub-dominant groups". In T. M. Pollard & S. B. Hyatt (Eds.), *Sex, Gender and Health* (pp. 137–161). Cambridge: Cambridge University Press.

Marshall, R. (1988). "Interpretation in doctor–patient interviews: A sociolinguistic analysis". *Culture, Medicine and Psychiatry, 12*, 201–218.

Martinic, S. (1996). *Organización de las conversaciones en contextos de ayuda social. El caso de un consultorio médico en barrio popular*. Ponencia presentada al Congreso Internacional "Cidade e educacao na Cultura pela paz", Rio de Janeiro, 4–6 Septiembre.

Maynard, D. W. (1991). "Interaction and asymmetry in clinical discourse". *American Journal of Sociology, 97*, 448–495.

Maynard, D. W. (1992). "On clinicians co-implicating recipients' perspective in the delivery of diagnostic news". In P. Drew & J. Heritage (Eds.), *Talk at Work: Interaction in Institutional Settings* (pp. 331–358). Cambridge: Cambridge University Press.

McCann, S., & J. Weinman (1996). "Encouraging patient participation in general practice consultations: Effects on consultation length and content, patient satisfaction and health". *Psychology and Health, 11* (6), 857–869.

McKenzie, P. (2002). "Communication barriers and information-seeking counterstrategies in accounts of practitioner–patient encounters". *Library and Information Science Research, 24*, 31–47.

Mishler, E. G. (1984). *The Discourse of Medicine. Dialectics in Medical Interviews*. Norwood, NJ: Ablex.

Molotch, H. L., & D. Boden (1985). "Talking social structure: Discourse, domination and the Watergate Hearings". *American Sociological Review, 50* (June), 273–288.

Morris, P. (1994). *The Bakhtin Reader: Selected Writings of Bakhtin, Medvedev, and Voloshinov*. London: E. Arnold.

Mulholland, J. (1994). "Multiple directives in the doctor–patient consultation". *Australian Journal of Communication, 21* (2), 74–85.

Muñoz, J. (1981). "Difficulties of a Hispanic American psychotherapist in the treatment of Hispanic American patients". *American Journal of Orthopsychiatry, 51*, 646–653.

Navarro, V. (1990). "Race or class versus race and class: Mortality differentials in the United States". *Lancet, 336*, 1238–1240.

Neighbour, R. (1987). *The Inner Consultation*. Newbury: Petroc Press.

Norrick, R. N. (1997). "Twice-told tales: Collaborative narration of familiar stories". *Language in Society, 26*, 199–220.

Ochs, E. (1979). "Transcription as theory". In E. Ochs & B. B. Schieffelin (Eds.), *Developmental Pragmatics* (pp. 43–72). New York: Academic Press.

Ochs, E., C. Taylor, D. Rudolph, & R. Smith (1992). "Storytelling as a theory-building activity". *Discourse Processes, 15*, 37–72.

Ong, L. M. L., J. C. J. M. De Haes, A. M. Hoos, & F. B. Lammes (1995). "Doctor–patient communication: A review of the literature". *Social Science and Medicine, 40* (7), 903–918.

Parrott, R. (1994). "Clarifying boundary-conditions and extending the motives for nonimmediate language use: A proposed model and test using physicians role experiences and gender". *Discourse Processes, 17*, 353–376.

Parrott, R., J. K. Burgoon, M. Burgoon, & B. A. LePoire (1989). "Privacy between physicians and patients: More than a matter of confidentiality". *Social Science and Medicine, 29* (12), 1381–1385.

Parsons, T. (1951). *The Social System*. New York: The Free Press.

Pauwels, A. (Ed.). (1987). *Women and Language in Australia and New Zealand Society*. Sydney: Australian Professional Publications.

Pauwels, A. (1995). *Cross-Cultural Communication in the Health Sciences: Communicating with Migrant Patients*. South Melbourne: Macmillan Education.

Pendleton, D. A., & S. Bochner (1980). "The communication of medical information in general practice consultations as a function of patients' social class". *Social Science and Medicine, 14A*, 669–673.

Polanyi, L. (1989). *Telling the American Story: A Structural and Cultural Analysis of Conversational Storytelling*. Boston: MIT Press.

Pollard, T. M., & S. B. Hyatt (1999). *Sex, Gender and Health*. Cambridge: Cambridge University Press.

Pomerantz, A. (1992). "Pursuing a response". In P. Drew & J. Heritage (Eds.), *Talk at Work: Interaction in Institutional Settings* (pp. 152–163). Cambridge: Cambridge University Press.

Pons, H., & J. L. Samaniego (1998). "Marcadores pragmáticos de apoyo discursivo en el habla culta de Santiago de Chile". *Onomázein: Revista de Lingüística, Filología y Traducción del Instituto de Letras de la Pontificia Universidad Católica de Chile, 3*, 11–25.

Prieto-Castillo, D. (1999). *El juego discursivo. Manual de análisis de estrategias discursivas*. Buenos Aires: Lumen Humanitas.

Prince, C. D. (1986). "Hablando con el doctor: Communication Problem between Doctors". Unpublished doctoral dissertation, Stanford University.

Quesada, G. (1976). "Language and communication barriers for health delivery to a minority group". *Social Science and Medicine, 10*, 323–327.

Randall, C. (1988). "Theoretical continuities in Goffman's work". In P. Drew & A. Wootton (Eds.), *Erving Goffman: Exploring the Interaction Order* (pp. 41–63). Abingdon: Polity Press.

Rehbein, J. (1980). "Sequentielles Erzählen – Erzählstrukturen von Immigranten bei Sozialberatungen in England". In K. Ehlich (Ed.), *Erzählen in Alltag*. Frankfurt a.M.: Suhrkamp.

Rehbein, J. (1994). "Rejective proposals: Semi-professional speech and clients' varieties in intercultural doctor–patient communication". *Multilingua: Journal of Cross-Cultural and Interlanguage Communication, 13*, 83–130.

Roter, D. (2000). "The enduring and evolving nature of the patient–physician relationship". *Patient Education and Counseling, 39*, 5–15.

Roter, D., J. Hall, & N. Katz (1987). "Relations between physicians' behaviors and analogue patients' satisfaction, recall and impressions". *Medical Care, 25* (5), 437–451.

Roter D., & J. Hall (1992). *Doctors Talking with Patients / Patients Talking with Doctors. Improving Communication in Medical Visits*. Westport, CT: Auburn House.

Royster, L. (1990). "Doctor–Patient Communication: An Exploration of Language Use During the Informed Consent". Unpublished doctoral dissertation, University of Pennsylvania.

Rozholdova, N. (1999). "No questions, please, we are doctors". *ESP Spectrum, 17* (Spring), 11–16.

Sacks, H. (1965–1971). Unpublished lectures notes. Los Angeles: University of California.

Sacks, H., E. Schegloff, & G. Jefferson (1974). "A simplest systematics for the organization of turn-taking for conversation". *Language, 50*, 696–735.

Salazar, S. L. (1978). *Avanzando: Gramática española y lectura*. New York: John Wiley.

Sarangi, S. (2001). "On demarcating the space between 'lay expertise' and 'expert laity'". *Text: An Interdisciplinary Journal for the Study of Discourse, 21*, 3–11.

Scarpaci, J. (1988). "Help-seeking behaviour, use, and satisfaction among frequent primary care users in Santiago de Chile". *Journal of Health and Social Behaviour, 29*, 199–213.

Schegloff, E. (1984). "On some questions and ambiguities in conversation". In M. Atkinson & J. Heritage (Eds.), *Structures of Social Action: Studies in Conversational Analysis* (pp. 28–52). Cambridge: Cambridge University Press.

Schiffrin, D. (1984). "Jewish argument as sociability". *Language in Society, 13*, 311–335.

Searle, J. R. (1969). *Speech Acts: An Essay in the Philosophy of Language*. London: Cambridge University Press.

Seijo, R., H. Gomez, & J. Freidenberg (1991). "Language as a communication barrier in medical care for Hispanic patients". *Hispanic Journal of Behavioral Sciences, 13*, 363–376.

Servicio Nacional de la Mujer. Dpto. Estudio y Estadísticas (2003). *Hombres y mujeres: Cómo ven hoy su rol en la sociedad y en la familia.* Santiago.

Shuy, R. (1983). "Three types of interferences to an effective exchange of information in the medical interview". In S. Fisher & A. D. Todd (Eds.), *The Social Organization of Doctor–Patient Communication* (pp. 17–30). Washington, DC: Center for Applied Linguistics Press.

Silverman, D. (1987). *Communication and Medical Practice.* London: Sage.

Sinclair, J., & R. M. Coulthard (1975). *Towards an Analysis of Discourse.* Oxford: Oxford University Press.

Smith, David C. (1997). "De-militarizing language". *Peace Magazine* 13 (July–August). <www.peacemagazine.org> (accessed April 2004)

Spiers, J. (1998). "The use of face work and politeness theory". *Qualitative Heath Research, 8,* 25–47.

Stearns, N., & D. M. Ross (1993). "Changing patterns of doctor–patient communication: The patient perspective". *Quality Life Research, 2,* 50.

Stevenson, F. A., C. A. Barry, N. Britten, & C. P. Bradley (2000). "Doctor–patient communication about drugs: The evidence for shared decision making". *Social Science and Medicine, 50* (6), 829–840.

Stivers, T., & J. Heritage (2001). "Breaking the sequential mold: Answering 'more than the question' during comprehensive history taking". *Text: An Interdisciplinary Journal for Discourse Research, 21,* 151–185.

Stoudemire, A. (Ed.). (1994). *Clinical Psychiatry for Medical Students.* Philadelphia: J. B. Lippincott.

Stubbs, M. (1983). *Discourse Analysis: The Sociolinguistic Analysis of Natural Language.* Oxford: Basil Blackwell.

Sundquist, J. (1995). "Ethnicity, social class and health. A population-based study on the influence of social factors on self-reported illness in 223 Latin American refugees, 333 Finnish and 126 South European labour migrants and 841 Swedish controls". *Social Science and Medicine, 40* (6), 777–787.

Tannen, D. (1983). "'I take out the rock-Dok!': How Greek women tell about being molested (and create involvement)". *Anthropological Linguistics, 25,* 359–374.

Tannen, D. (1984). *Conversational Style: Analyzing Talk Among Friends.* Norwood, NJ: Ablex.

Tannen, D. (1987). *Power Through Discourse.* Norwood, NJ: Ablex.

Tannen, D. (1989). *Talking Voices: Repetition, Dialogue, and Imagery in Conversational Discourse.* Cambridge: Cambridge University Press.

Tannen, D. (1993). "What's in a frame? Surface evidence for underlying expectations". In D. Tannen (Ed.), *Framing in Discourse* (pp. 14–56). New York: Oxford University Press.

Tannen, D., & C. Wallat (1993). "Interactive frames and knowledge schemas in interaction: Examples from a medical examination/interview". In D. Tannen (Ed.), *Framing in Discourse* (pp. 57–76). New York: Oxford University Press.

Ten Have, P. (1991). "Talk and institution: A reconsideration of the 'asymmetry' of doctor–patient interaction". In D. Boden & D. H. Zimmerman (Eds.), *Talk and Social Structure: Studies in Ethnomethodology and Conversation Analysis* (pp. 138–163). Cambridge: Polity Press.

Thompson, C., & L. Pledger (1993). "Doctor–patient communication: Is patient knowledge of medical terminology improving?" *Health Communication, 5*, 89–97.

Thompson, T. (1998). "Patient/health professional communication". In L. Jackson & B. K. Duffy (Eds.), *Health Communication Research: A Guide to Developments and Directions* (pp. 37–56). Westport, CT: Greenwood.

Thorne, S. E., K. T. Nyhlin, & B. L. Paterson (2000). "Attitudes toward patient expertise in chronic illness". *International Journal of Nursing Studies, 37*, 303–311.

Todd, A. D. (1993). "A diagnosis of doctor–patient discourse in the prescription of contraception". In A. D. Todd & S. Fisher (Eds.), *The Social Organization of Doctor–Patient Communication* (pp. 183–212). Norwood, NJ: Ablex.

Todd, A. D., & S. Fisher (Eds.). (1988). *Gender and Discourse: The Power of Talk*. Norwood, NJ: Ablex.

Todd, A. D., & S. Fisher (Eds.). (1993). *The Social Organization of Doctor–Patient Communication*. Norwood, NJ: Ablex. [Rev. ed. of Fisher & Todd 1983]

Tran, A., P. Haidet, R. L. Street Jr., K. J. O'Malley, F. Martin, & C. M. Ashton (in press). "Empowering communication: A community-based intervention for patients". *Patient Education and Counseling.*

Triandis, H. C., G. Marín, J. Lisanky, & H. Betancourt (1984). "*Simpatía* as a cultural script of Hispanics". *Journal of Personality and Social Psychology, 47* (6), 1363–1375.

Trosborg, A. (1987). "Apology strategies in natives/non-natives". *Journal of Pragmatics, 11*, 147–167.

van Dijk, T. A. (1982). "Episodes as units of discourse analysis". In D. Tannen (Ed.), *Analysing Discourse: Text and Talk* (pp. 177–195). Washington: Georgetown University Press.

van Dijk, T. A. (1987). *Communicating Racism: Ethnic Prejudice in Thought and Talk*. Newbury Park, CA: Sage.

van Dijk, T. A. (1995a). "Discourse semantics and ideology". *Discourse and Society, 5*, 243–289.

van Dijk, T. A. (1995b). *Prensa, racismo y poder*. [Cuadernos del posgrado en comunicación]. Mexico: Universidad Iberoamericana.

van Dijk, T. A. (1996). "Discourse, power and access". In C. R. Caldas-Coulthard & M. Coulthard (Eds.), *Texts and Practices: Readings in Critical Discourse Analyisis* (pp. 84–104). London: Routledge.

van Dijk, T. A. (Ed.). (1997a). *Discourse as Structure and Process*. [Discourse Studies: A Multidisciplinary Introduction 1]. London: Sage.

van Dijk, T. A. (Ed.). (1997b). *Discourse as Social Interaction*. [Discourse Studies: A Multidisciplinary Introduction 2]. London: Sage.

von Raffler-Engel, W. (1989). *Doctor–Patient Interaction*. Amsterdam: John Benjamins.

Waitzkin, H. (1983). *The Second Sickness*. New York: The Free Press.

Waitzkin, H. (1985). "Information given in medical care". *Journal of Health and Social Behavior, 26*, 81–101.

Walker, K. L., C. L. Arnold, M. Miller-Day, & L. M. Webb (2002). "Investigating the physician–patient relationship: examining emerging themes". *Health Communication, 14*, 45–68.

Wallen, J., H. Waitzkin, & J. D. Stoeckle (1979). "Physician stereotypes about female health and illness". *Women and Health, 4*, 135–146.

Weitzman, P. F., & E. A. Weitzman (2003). "Promoting communication with older adults: Protocol for resolving interpersonal conflicts and for enhancing interactions with doctors". *Clinical Psychology Review, 23*, 523–535.

Welch Cline, R. (2003). "At the intersection of micro and macro: Opportunities and challenges for physician–patient communication research". *Patient Education and Counseling, 50*, 13–16.

West, C. (1984). *Routine Complications: Troubles with Talk between Doctors and Patients.* Bloomington: Indiana University Press.

West, C. (1990). "Not just 'doctors' orders': Directives–response sequences in patients' visits to women and men physicians". *Discourse and Society, 1*, 85–112.

West, C., & D., & Zimmerman (1991). "Doing gender". In J. Lorber & S. Farrell (Eds.), *The Social Construction of Gender* (pp. 1–29). Newbury Park, CA: Sage.

White, D. R., H. B. Muss, R. Michielutte, M. K. Cooper, D. V. Jackson, F. Richards, J. J. Stuart, & C. L. Spurr (1984). "Informed consent: Patient information forms in chemotherapy trials". *American Journal of Clinical Oncology, 17*, 183–190.

Williams, S., J. Weinman, & J. Dale (1998). "Doctor–patient communication and patient satisfaction: A review". *Family Practice, 15* (5), 480–492.

Winter, J. (1992). "The meaning and pragmatics of difference". *Working Papers on Language, Gender and Sexism, 18*, 77–186.

Winter, J., & G. Wigglesworth (1993). "Language and gender: A case study of applied linguistics in Australia". *Australian Review of Applied Linguistics, Series S* (10), 1–12.

Wodak, R. (Ed.). (1989). *Language, Power and Ideology: Studies in Political Discourse.* Amsterdam: John Benjamins.

Wodak, R. (1995). "Critical linguistics and critical discourse analysis". In J. Verschueren, J.-A. Östman, & J. Blommaert (Eds.), *Handbook of Pragmatics: Manual* (pp. 204–210). Amsterdam: John Benjamins.

Wodak, R. (1996). *Disorders of Discourse.* London: Longman.

Wodak, R. (1997). "Introduction: Some important issues in the study of gender and discourse". In R. Wodak (Ed.), *Gender and Discourse* (pp. 1–20). London: Sage.

Wodk, R. (1999a). "Critical discourse analysis at the end of the 20th century". *Research on Language and Social Interaction, 32*, 185–193.

Wodak, R. (1999b). "Discourse and racism: European perspectives". *Annual Review of Anthropology, 28*, 175–199.

Wodak, R., & B. Matouschek (1993). "'We are dealing with people whose origins one can clearly tell just by looking': Critical discourse analysis and the study of neo-racism in contemporary Austria". *Discourse and Society, 4*, 225–248.

Working Party (1997). *From Compliance to Concordance: Achieving Shared Goals in Medicine Taking.* [Report of the Working Party]. London: Royal Pharmaceutical Society of Great Britain; Merck, Sharp and Dohme.

Yáñez, S. (1999). "Consideraciones sobre flexibilidad laboral planteadas desde una mirada de género". In J. & S. Yáñez (Eds.), *Sindicalismo, género y flexibilización en el Mercosur y Chile. Inserción laboral femenina.* Santiago: Fundación Friedrich Ebert/CEM.

Zimmerman, D. H., & C. West (1975). "Sex roles, interruptions and silences in conversations". In B. Thorne & N. Henley (Eds.), *Language and Sex: Difference and Dominance* (pp. 105–129). Rowley, MA: Newbury House.

Appendices

Appendix 1

Aproximate total word count of doctors and patients

Dyad	Doctor	Word Count	Patient	Word Count
Consultation 1 FD–FP	Ana	1,019	Alicia	1,017
Consultation 2 FD–FP	Ana	323	Beatriz	307
Consultation 3 FD–FP	Ana	874	Carmen	1,292
Consultation 4 FD–MP	Ana	1,684	David	791
Consultation 5 FD–MP	Ana	338	Esteban	305
Consultation 6 FD–MP	Ana	961	Flavio	592
Consultation 7 FD–FP	Berta	150	Gina	171
Consultation 8 FD–FP	Berta	564	Hilda	636
Consultation 9 FD–FP	Berta	222	Javiera	280
Consultation 10 MD–MP	Carlos	756	Leonel	664
Consultation 11 MD–MP	Carlos	871	Manuel	625
Consultation 12 MD–MP	Carlos	842	Nicolás	929
Consultation 13 MD–FP	Carlos	1,871	Olga	1,285
Consultation 14 MD–FP	Carlos	230	Paola	404
Consultation 15 MD–FP	Carlos	840	Rosa	1,000

Dyad	Doctor	Word Count	Patient	Word Count
Consultation 16 MD–MP	Daniel	50	Samuel	79
Consultation 17 MD–MP	Daniel	143	Tito	368
Consultation 18 MD–MP	Daniel	198	Victor	281
Consultation 19 MD–FP	Daniel	170	Wilma	105
Consultation 20 MD–FP	Daniel	72	Ximena	642
Consultation 21 MD–FP	Daniel	513	Yolanda	846
Consultation 22 MD–FP	Daniel	138	Zenobia	304
Total number of words:		12,829		12,923

FD = Female doctor   FP = Female patient
MD = Male doctor   MP = Male patient

Appendix 2a (English version)

PATIENT QUESTIONNAIRE

Name of Project: "Doctor and patient discourse in Chile: A social interactive investigation"

Date:

Please make a cross ☒ where appropriate

Sex

Female ☐ Male ☐

Nationality: ______________________

Age

In which category are you?

20–25 ☐
26–30 ☐
31–35 ☐
36–40 ☐
41–45 ☐
46–50 ☐
51–55 ☐
56–60 ☐

Other ______________________

Occupation: ______________________

How many times (approximately) have you visited the same doctor before?

2–4 ☐
4–6 ☐

For how long have you visited the same doctor?

less than a year ☐
a year ☐
over a year ☐
over two years ☐
over three years ☐

Other ______________________

What do you like from a doctor? (leave ample space to write down patients' ideas)

What you dislike from a doctor? (leave ample space to write down patients' ideas)

Appendix 2b (Spanish version)

CUESTIONARIO PARA EL PACIENTE

Nombre del proyecto: «El discurso hablado del médico y el paciente en Chile: Una investigación social interactiva»

Fecha:

Por favor marque con una cruz ☒

Sexo
Femenino ☐ Masculino ☐

Nacionalidad: ______________________

Edad

¿En qué categoría de edad se encuentra Ud.?

20–25 ☐
26–30 ☐
31–35 ☐
36–40 ☐
41–45 ☐
46–50 ☐
51–55 ☐
56–60 ☐

Otra ______________________

Actividad: ______________________

¿Cuántas veces (aproximadamente) ha visitado al mismo médico?

2–4 ☐
4–6 ☐

¿Hace cuánto tiempo que visita al mismo médico?

menos de un año ☐
un año ☐
más de un año ☐
más de dos años ☐
más de tres años ☐

Otro ______________________

¿Qué le gusta de un médico? (dejar bastante espacio para la respuesta de los pacientes)

¿Qué no le gusta de un médico? (dejar bastante espacio para la respuesta de los pacientes)

Appendix 3a (English version)

DOCTOR QUESTIONNAIRE

Name of the Project: "Doctor and patient discourse in Chile: A social interactive investigation"

Date:

Please make a cross ☒ where appropriate

Sex

Female ☐ Male ☐

Nationality: ______________________________

Age

In which category are you?

20–25 ☐	41–45 ☐
26–30 ☐	46–50 ☐
31–35 ☐	51–55 ☐
36–40 ☐	56–60 ☐

Other ______________________________

How many years' practice in medicine do you have?

Appendix 3b (Spanish version)

CUESTIONARIO PARA EL MEDICO

Nombre del proyecto: «El discurso hablado del médico y el paciente en Chile: una investigación social interactiva»

Fecha:

Por favor marque con una cruz ☒

Sexo

Femenino ☐ Masculino ☐

Nacionalidad: ______________________________

Edad

¿En qué categoría de edad se encuentra Ud.?

20–25 ☐ 41–45 ☐
26–30 ☐ 46–50 ☐
31–35 ☐ 51–55 ☐
36–40 ☐ 56–60 ☐

Otra ______________________________

¿Cúantos años de experiencia médica tiene?

Appendix 4

Symbols used in discourse transcriptions

Unit	Spanish conventional last truncated syllable in *para* (*pa'*) and *pues* (*po'*)	'
	Truncated syllable (middle and final)	–
Speakers	Speaker identity/turn start	:
	Speech overlap	[ ]
	Latching	=
Transitional continuity	Final	.
	Continuing	,
	Appeal	¿ ?
	Exclamation	¡ !
Tone	Fall	\
	Rise	/
	Loud voice	CAPITAL LETTERS
Pause	Long	... (N)
	Medium	...
	Short	..
Vocal Noises	Inhalation	(H)
	Exhalation	(Hx)
Quality voice	Emphasis	CAPITAL LETTERS
	Laugh quality	<@ @>
	Whisper	<WH WH>
Lengthening	Vowel elongation	:
Transcriber's perspective	Researcher's comment	(( ))
	Uncertain hearing	<X X>
Specialized notations	False start	< >
	Doctor's speech	D
	Patient's speech	P

The symbols of transcription used in this study correspond to Du Bois (1991). Adaptations have been made to accommodate Spanish data.

Appendix 5a (English version)

EXPLANATORY STATEMENT FOR PATIENT AND DOCTOR

The following pages briefly describe the project.

ANY INFORMATION GIVEN IS STRICTLY CONFIDENTIAL

The title of this research is: "Doctor and patient discourse in Chile: A social interactive investigation".

The researcher is Dr. Marisa Cordella, who comes from Monash University, Melbourne, Australia. She will be involved with those who are willing to participate in this study and she will give you further information about the research if you so wish.

What is the aim of this research?

The aim of this research is to understand how doctors and patients communicate during a consultation. The conversation between both of you will be tape-recorded and later analysed according to current linguistic theories.

What are you required to do?

Patients will be asked to complete a questionnaire before the consultation. Doctors will be interviewed before the start of the day's session. The conversation between patient and doctor will be recorded provided they have agreed and signed the consent form.

How long should it take?

You will be required to participate in this study for the length of the consultation with an additional 5 minutes to complete the questionnaire.

Can I refuse to participate in this study?

YOU ARE FREE to participate in it. Your refusal or withdrawal from the tape recording **will not affect you in any way**. You have the right to withdraw your consent to participate at **any** time. You also have the right to listen to your recording and withdraw your consent if you wish.

CONFIDENTIALITY?

YOUR CONTRIBUTION IS STRICTLY CONFIDENTIAL

No one will have access to the data except the researcher. Original names will not be included in any transcript or publication. The data will be kept under lock and key. Nothing which could identify an individual person will be released. The information will not go into the participant's medical record.

What should I do if I have queries or if I would like to have more information about it?

Further information can be sought at any time from Dr. Marisa Cordella, who will be in the clinic during the recording. You can also write to her in Australia if doubts and queries come to mind after the completion of recordings in Chile, or send a letter to Dr. Joanne Winter at Monash University, Melbourne, Australia to ask for further information.

Dr. Marisa Cordella (I will get an address from Chile as well)
Monash University
Department of Romance Languages
Spanish Section
Wellington Road
CLAYTON VIC 3168
AUSTRALIA

Dr. Joanne Winter
Monash University
Department of Linguistics
Spanish Section
Wellington Road
CLAYTON VIC 3168
AUSTRALIA

Can I have access to the results?

Interested participants (doctors and patients) will be informed of the final results. Copies of the thesis and articles emanating from this work will be sent to the hospital. Please note that the time allocated for this study is around 6 years so results are unlikely to be ready before that date.

What should I do if I have a complaint about this study?

Should you have any complaint concerning the manner in which this research is being conducted, please do not hesitate to contact: The Standing Committee on Ethics in Research on Humans at the following address:

The Secretary
The Standing Committee on Ethics in Research on Humans
Monash University, Wellington Road, Clayton, Victoria 3168
Telephone (03) 990 52052 Fax: (03) 990 53866

At the end of the recording you will receive a small present to thank you for your co-operation.

Appendix 5b (Spanish version)

DECLARACIÓN ACLARATORIA PARA PACIENTE Y MEDICO

Las siguientes páginas describen brevemente este proyecto.

TODA INFORMACIÓN QUE UD. ENTREGUE SERÁ MATERIAL ESTRICTAMENTE CONFIDENCIAL

El título de esta investigación es: «El discurso hablado del médico y el paciente en Chile: una investigación social interactiva».

La investigadora es la Dra. Marisa Cordella proveniente de la Universidad de Monash de Melbourne, Australia. Ella le entregará información sobre la investigación y estará junto a los participantes que deseen contribuir en el estudio.

¿Cuál es el objetivo de este estudio?

El objetivo de esta investigación es el entender cómo el discurso entre el médico y el paciente se desarrolla durante la consulta médica. La conversación entre Uds. dos se grabará, transcribirá, y luego analizará siguiendo las teorías actuales de lingüística.

¿Qué cosa se requiere de Ud.?

Se les pedirá a los pacientes que llenen un cuestionario antes de la consulta. A los médico se les entrevistará antes de comenzar la sesión del día y la conversación entre ambos (paciente y médico) se grabará si ambas partes han consentido.

¿Cuánto tiempo se requiere?

El tiempo que se requiere de los participantes es equivalente a la duración de la consulta, con un tiempo adicional de 5 minutos para completar el cuestionario.

¿Puedo rehusarme a participar?

UD. ESTA LIBRE EN PARTICIPAR EN ESTE ESTUDIO

Si Ud. no desea participar o si se arrepiente luego de haber consentido, esto **no le afectará en absoluto**. Ud. tiene el derecho de retirar su consentimiento de participación en **cualquier momento** e incluso puede escuchar la conversación una vez que se haya grabado y pedir que no se incluya en el estudio.

¿Confidencialidad?

CUALQUIER INFORMACIÓN QUE OTORGUE ES ESTRICTAMENTE CONFIDENCIAL

Sólo la investigadora tendrá acceso a los datos.

Los nombres originales de los participantes no se incluirán ni en las transcripciones ni en ninguna publicación. Toda la información se guardará bajo llave. Lo que se publique en el futuro no contendrá ninguna información que pueda descubrir la identidad de los participantes. Ningún tipo de información que Ud. haya dado en este estudio se incluirá en los registros médicos.

¿Qué debería hacer si me surgen dudas o si deseo obtener mayor información al respecto?

La Dra. Marisa Cordella quien estará en la clínica en el momento de la grabación puede darle mayor información sobre el proyecto en cualquier minuto que Ud. lo requiera. Ud. también puede enviarle una carta a Australia si tiene preguntas luego de haber completado las grabaciones en Chile. Ud. también puede escribirle a la Dra. Joanne Winter de la Universidad de Monash, Melbourne, Australia, si desea mayor información.

Dra. Marisa Cordella (Entregaré además una dirección en Chile)
Monash University
Department of Romance Languages
Spanish Section
Wellington Road
CLAYTON VIC 3168
AUSTRALIA

Dr. Joanne Winter
Monash University
Department of Linguistics
Wellington Road
CLAYTON VIC 3168
AUSTRALIA

¿Cómo podría tener acceso a los resultados?

Los participantes (médicos y pacientes) que estén interesados estarán al tanto de los resultados por intermedio de una copia de la tesis y de los artículos que se publicarán y que se enviarán al hospital. Tenga presente que el estudio durará alrededor de 6 años, por lo tanto será muy difícil tener resultados antes de esa fecha.

¿A quien debería contactar en caso que tuviera alguna queja sobre el desarrollo del estudio?

Si hubiera alguna queja con respecto a la forma en que la investigación se llevó a cabo, tenga la amabilidad de comunicarse con "El Comité Ético de Investigación con Seres Humanos", dirija su carta a la siguiente dirección:

The Secretary
The Standing Committee on Ethics in Research of Humans
Monash University
Wellington Road
CLAYTON VIC 3168
AUSTRALIA
Teléfono (03) 990 52052 Fax (03) 990 53866

Al final de la grabación Ud. recibirá un pequeño obsequio como forma de agradecimiento por su participación.

Appendix 6a (English version)

CONSENT FORM

I have read the explanatory statement and I agree to participate in the study "Doctor and patient discourse in Chile: A social interactive investigation".

Date: ____________________________________

Name: ____________________________________

Signature: ____________________________________

Appendix 6b (Spanish version)

CONSENTIMIENTO

He leído la nota explicativa y estoy de acuerdo en participar en el estudio "El discurso hablado del médico y el paciente en Chile: una investigación social interactiva".

Fecha: ________________________________

Nombre: ________________________________

Firma: ________________________________

Index

In the *Pragmatics & Beyond New Series* the following titles have been published thus far or are scheduled for publication:

78 **SELL, Roger D.:** Literature as Communication. The foundations of mediating criticism. 2000. xiv, 348 pp.

79 **ANDERSEN, Gisle and Thorstein FRETHEIM (eds.):** Pragmatic Markers and Propositional Attitude. 2000. viii, 273 pp.

80 **UNGERER, Friedrich (ed.):** English Media Texts – Past and Present. Language and textual structure. 2000. xiv, 286 pp.

81 **DI LUZIO, Aldo, Susanne GÜNTHNER and Franca ORLETTI (eds.):** Culture in Communication. Analyses of intercultural situations. 2001. xvi, 341 pp.

82 **KHALIL, Esam N.:** Grounding in English and Arabic News Discourse. 2000. x, 274 pp.

83 **MÁRQUEZ REITER, Rosina:** Linguistic Politeness in Britain and Uruguay. A contrastive study of requests and apologies. 2000. xviii, 225 pp.

84 **ANDERSEN, Gisle:** Pragmatic Markers and Sociolinguistic Variation. A relevance-theoretic approach to the language of adolescents. 2001. ix, 352 pp.

85 **COLLINS, Daniel E.:** Reanimated Voices. Speech reporting in a historical-pragmatic perspective. 2001. xx, 384 pp.

86 **IFANTIDOU, Elly:** Evidentials and Relevance. 2001. xii, 225 pp.

87 **MUSHIN, Ilana:** Evidentiality and Epistemological Stance. Narrative Retelling. 2001. xviii, 244 pp.

88 **BAYRAKTAROĞLU, Arın and Maria SIFIANOU (eds.):** Linguistic Politeness Across Boundaries. The case of Greek and Turkish. 2001. xiv, 439 pp.

89 **ITAKURA, Hiroko:** Conversational Dominance and Gender. A study of Japanese speakers in first and second language contexts. 2001. xviii, 231 pp.

90 **KENESEI, István and Robert M. HARNISH (eds.):** Perspectives on Semantics, Pragmatics, and Discourse. A Festschrift for Ferenc Kiefer. 2001. xxii, 352 pp.

91 **GROSS, Joan:** Speaking in Other Voices. An ethnography of Walloon puppet theaters. 2001. xxviii, 341 pp.

92 **GARDNER, Rod:** When Listeners Talk. Response tokens and listener stance. 2001. xxii, 281 pp.

93 **BARON, Bettina and Helga KOTTHOFF (eds.):** Gender in Interaction. Perspectives on femininity and masculinity in ethnography and discourse. 2002. xxiv, 357 pp.

94 **McILVENNY, Paul (ed.):** Talking Gender and Sexuality. 2002. x, 332 pp.

95 **FITZMAURICE, Susan M.:** The Familiar Letter in Early Modern English. A pragmatic approach. 2002. viii, 263 pp.

96 **HAVERKATE, Henk:** The Syntax, Semantics and Pragmatics of Spanish Mood. 2002. vi, 241 pp.

97 **MAYNARD, Senko K.:** Linguistic Emotivity. Centrality of place, the topic-comment dynamic, and an ideology of *pathos* in Japanese discourse. 2002. xiv, 481 pp.

98 **DUSZAK, Anna (ed.):** Us and Others. Social identities across languages, discourses and cultures. 2002. viii, 522 pp.

99 **JASZCZOLT, Katarzyna M. and Ken TURNER (eds.):** Meaning Through Language Contrast. Volume 1. 2003. xii, 388 pp.

100 **JASZCZOLT, Katarzyna M. and Ken TURNER (eds.):** Meaning Through Language Contrast. Volume 2. 2003. viii, 496 pp.

101 **LUKE, Kang Kwong and Theodossia-Soula PAVLIDOU (eds.):** Telephone Calls. Unity and diversity in conversational structure across languages and cultures. 2002. x, 295 pp.

102 **LEAFGREN, John:** Degrees of Explicitness. Information structure and the packaging of Bulgarian subjects and objects. 2002. xii, 252 pp.

103 **FETZER, Anita and Christiane MEIERKORD (eds.):** Rethinking Sequentiality. Linguistics meets conversational interaction. 2002. vi, 300 pp.

104 **BEECHING, Kate:** Gender, Politeness and Pragmatic Particles in French. 2002. x, 251 pp.

105 **BLACKWELL, Sarah E.:** Implicatures in Discourse. The case of Spanish NP anaphora. 2003. xvi, 303 pp.

106 **BUSSE, Ulrich:** Linguistic Variation in the Shakespeare Corpus. Morpho-syntactic variability of second person pronouns. 2002. xiv, 344 pp.

107 **TAAVITSAINEN, Irma and Andreas H. JUCKER (eds.):** Diachronic Perspectives on Address Term Systems. 2003. viii, 446 pp.

108 **BARRON, Anne:** Acquisition in Interlanguage Pragmatics. Learning how to do things with words in a study abroad context. 2003. xviii, 403 pp.

109 **MAYES, Patricia:** Language, Social Structure, and Culture. A genre analysis of cooking classes in Japan and America. 2003. xiv, 228 pp.

110 **ANDROUTSOPOULOS, Jannis K. and Alexandra GEORGAKOPOULOU (eds.):** Discourse Constructions of Youth Identities. 2003. viii, 343 pp.

111 **ENSINK, Titus and Christoph SAUER (eds.):** Framing and Perspectivising in Discourse. 2003. viii, 227 pp.

112 **LENZ, Friedrich (ed.):** Deictic Conceptualisation of Space, Time and Person. 2003. xiv, 279 pp.

113 **PANTHER, Klaus-Uwe and Linda L. THORNBURG (eds.):** Metonymy and Pragmatic Inferencing. 2003. xii, 285 pp.

114 **KÜHNLEIN, Peter, Hannes RIESER and Henk ZEEVAT (eds.):** Perspectives on Dialogue in the New Millennium. 2003. xii, 400 pp.

115 **KÄRKKÄINEN, Elise:** Epistemic Stance in English Conversation. A description of its interactional functions, with a focus on *I think*. 2003. xii, 213 pp.

116 **GRANT, Colin B. (ed.):** Rethinking Communicative Interaction. New interdisciplinary horizons. 2003. viii, 330 pp.

117 **WU, Ruey-Jiuan Regina:** Stance in Talk. A conversation analysis of Mandarin final particles. 2004. xvi, 260 pp.

118 **CHENG, Winnie:** Intercultural Conversation. 2003. xii, 279 pp.

119 **HILTUNEN, Risto and Janne SKAFFARI (eds.):** Discourse Perspectives on English. Medieval to modern. 2003. viii, 243 pp.

120 **AIJMER, Karin and Anna-Brita STENSTRÖM (eds.):** Discourse Patterns in Spoken and Written Corpora. 2004. viii, 279 pp.

121 **FETZER, Anita:** Recontextualizing Context. Grammaticality meets appropriateness. 2004. x, 272 pp.

122 **GONZÁLEZ, Montserrat:** Pragmatic Markers in Oral Narrative. The case of English and Catalan. 2004. xvi, 410 pp.

123 **MÁRQUEZ REITER, Rosina and María Elena PLACENCIA (eds.):** Current Trends in the Pragmatics of Spanish. 2004. xvi, 383 pp.

124 **VINE, Bernadette:** Getting Things Done at Work. The discourse of power in workplace interaction. 2004. x, 278 pp.

125 **LERNER, Gene H. (ed.):** Conversation Analysis. Studies from the first generation. 2004. x, 302 pp.

126 **WU, Yi'an:** Spatial Demonstratives in English and Chinese. Text and Cognition. xviii, 236 pp. *Expected Fall 2004*

127 **BRISARD, Frank, Michael MEEUWIS and Bart VANDENABEELE (eds.):** Seduction, Community, Speech. A Festschrift for Herman Parret. vi, 196 pp. + index. *Expected Fall 2004*

128 **CORDELLA, Marisa:** The Dynamic Consultation. A discourse analytical study of doctor–patient communication. 2004. xii, 252 pp.

129 **TABOADA, María Teresa:** Building Coherence and Cohesion. Task-oriented dialogue in English and Spanish. xvii, 244 pp. + index. *Expected Fall 2004*

130 **HALMARI, Helena and Tuija VIRTANEN (eds.):** Persuasion Across Genres. A linguistic approach. viii, 244 pp. + index. *Expected Fall 2004*

131 **JANOSCHKA, Anja:** Web Advertising. New forms of communication on the Internet. xiv, 221 pp. + index. *Expected Winter 04-05*

132 **ONODERA, Noriko:** Japanese Discourse Markers. Synchronic and diachronic discourse analysis. xiv, 240 pp. + index. *Expected Winter 04-05*

A complete list of titles in this series can be found on the publishers website, **www.benjamins.com**